Accountability in Nursing Practice

Accountability in Nursing Practice

Edited by

Roger Watson

Senior Lecturer at the Department of Nursing Studies
The University of Edinburgh
Scotland, UK

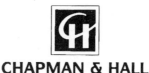

CHAPMAN & HALL

London · Glasgow · Weinheim · New York · Tokyo · Melbourne · Madras

Published by Chapman & Hall, 2–6 Boundary Row, London SE1 8HN, UK

Chapman & Hall, 2–6 Boundary Row, London SE1 8HN, UK

Blackie Academic & Professional, Wester Cleddens Road, Bishopbriggs, Glasgow G64 2NZ, UK

Chapman & Hall GmbH, Pappelallee 3, 69469 Weinheim, Germany

Chapman & Hall USA, 115 Fifth Avenue, New York NY 10003, USA

Chapman & Hall Japan, ITP-Japan, Kyowa Building, 3F, 2-2-1 Hirakawacho, Chiyoda-ku, Tokyo 102, Japan

Chapman & Hall Australia, 102 Dodds Street, South Melbourne, Victoria 3205, Australia

Chapman & Hall India, R. Seshadri, 32 Second Main Road, CIT East, Madras 600 035, India

Distributed in the USA and Canada by Singular Publishing Group Inc., 4284 41st Street, San Diego, California 92105

First edition 1995

© 1995 Chapman & Hall

Typeset in Times 10/12pt by Saxon Graphics Ltd, Derby
Printed in England by Clays Ltd, St Ives plc

ISBN 0 412 49860 X   1 56593 172 6 (USA)

A catalogue record for this book is available from the British Library

Library of Congress Catalog Card Number: 95-69208

∞   Printed on permanent acid-free text paper, manufactured in accordance with ANSI/NISO Z39. 48-1992 and ANSI/NISO Z39.48-1984 (Permanence of Paper).

Contents

List of contributors   vii

Part One BACKGROUND

1 **Introduction: accountability in nursing**   1
Roger Watson
2 **The development of nursing as an accountable profession**   18
Susan McGann

Part Two DELIVERY OF CARE

3 **Accountability in nursing models and the nursing process**   33
Helen Chalmers
4 **Standards of care, quality assurance and accountability**   49
Lesley Duff
5 **Accountability in primary nursing**   70
Sheila Rodgers

Part Three AREAS OF PRACTICE

6 **Where does the buck stop? Accountability in midwifery**   95
Rosemary Mander
7 **Accounts, accounting and accountability in psychiatric nursing**   107
Stephen Tilley
8 **Accountability in community nursing**   131
Sarah Baggaley and Alison Bryans
9 **Working with children: accountability and paediatric nursing**   147
Gosia Brykczynska

Part Four LEGAL AND ETHICAL ISSUES

10 **The legal accountability of the nurse**   163
John H. Tingle
11 **Accountability – the ethical dimension**   177
Kath Melia

12 Accountability in life and death decisions 181
Hazel McHaffie

Part Five RESEARCH AND EDUCATION

13 Accountability in nursing research 209
Alison J. Tierney
14 Accountability in nursing education 232
Diane Marks-Maran

References 241

Index 255

Contributors

Sarah Baggaley
BSc SRN SCM HV
Lecturer, Department of Nursing Studies, University of Edinburgh

Alison Bryans
BA MSc RGN HV RNT
Research Fellow/Lecturer, Department of Nursing and Community Health,
   Glasgow Caledonian University

Gosia Brykczynska
RGN RSCN BA BSc CertED CertOncNurs DiplPH
Lecturer in Ethics and Philosophy, Royal College of Nursing, London

Helen Chalmers
BA RGN DipN(London)
Nurse Educationist, Bath

Lesley Duff
Research and Development Officer, Dynamic Quality Improvement
   Programme, Royal College of Nursing, London

Rosemary Mander
MSc PhD RGN SCM MTD
Senior Lecturer, Department of Nursing Studies, University of Edinburgh

Diane Marks-Maran
Vice-Principal, Queen Charlotte's College of Health and Science, Thames
   Valley University

Susan McGann
BA (Hons) Dip Archival Studies
Archivist, Royal College of Nursing, Edinburgh

Hazel McHaffie
PhD SRN RM
Institute of Medical Ethics, Department of Medicine, Edinburgh University,
  Royal Infirmary of Edinburgh

Kath Melia
BNurs PhD
Senior Lecturer, Head of Department, Department of Nursing Studies,
  University of Edinburgh

Sheila Rodgers
BSc MSc RGN
Lecturer, Department of Nursing Studies, University of Edinburgh

Alison J. Tierney
BSc RGN PhD
Reader (formerly Director of the Nursing Research Unit), Department
  of Nursing Studies, University of Edinburgh

Stephen Tilley
BA PhD RMN
Lecturer, Department of Nursing Studies, University of Edinburgh

John H. Tingle
BA Law Hons, Cert Ed, MEd
Barrister, Health Care Risks Solutions Reader in Health Law, Director, Centre
  for Health Law, Nottingham Law School, Nottingham Trent University

Roger Watson
BSc PhD RGN CBiol MIBiol
Senior Lecturer, Department of Nursing Studies, University of Edinburgh

PART ONE

Background

Introduction: accountability in nursing

Roger Watson

INTRODUCTION

The literature on accountability as a concept in nursing has been growing steadily for the past two decades. Lewis and Batey's (1982a,b) articles on the subject reviewed literature from the mid-1970s and greatly clarified some of the issues. The seminal nature of Lewis and Batey's work is exemplified by the present volume, in which almost every author makes reference to their work.

More recently, the United Kingdom Central Council for Nursing, Midwifery and Health Visiting (UKCC 1989) has produced a succinct document which was aimed at the profession in the United Kingdom and which greatly helped to put the issue to the forefront of thinking among British nurses. In so doing, the UKCC succeeded in stimulating much thinking, both within and outwith the profession, on the legal, ethical and practical consequences for individual nurses of assuming accountability and being accountable.

The nature of accountability

The question is immediately raised of the scope of accountability in nursing, its nature and the directions in which it goes. This volume was commissioned to bring together a wide variety of writers, most of whom were nurses, in order to present their thinking on the issue of accountability as it applies in a number of different nursing situations. It also includes significant chapters on the historical development of accountability in nursing, and its legal and ethical implications.

Many of the authors expressed concern that the issue would be adequately and exhaustively covered in chapters other than their own, and that they would not have much left to say. They were nevertheless encouraged to address the issue without recourse to worries about what others might say, and to investigate accountability as it impinged on their specific areas of nursing, whether they were working with children or the mentally ill, for example, or in the community. Readers may judge the result for themselves, but I wish to point out that very little in the original manuscripts required to be changed. I am uncertain what this tells us about accountability as a concept, other than that it is, at the very least, 'hydra-headed' – it appears to mean slightly different things to different people in the profession. However, the material which was common to a number of chapters could not be removed, as each author approached the subject in a unique way and used the concept differently in order to exemplify how it guided practice in their particular field.

The problem of accountability is not unique to nursing. The advent of health service reforms, with the introduction of the purchaser–provider concept of services, has raised the issue of accountability in the health service generally. Knowles (1994), while explaining that the reforms did not necessarily create a market in the NHS, stated that they have demanded 'explicitness and transparency in health-care purchasing decisions' and, with reference to this volume, it is inevitable that this is putting pressure on nursing to be more accountable. Prentice (1994) states that 'there is no precise definition of 'accountability', but goes on to say that 'It is about answering, responsiveness, openness...not to mention participation and obedience to external laws'. It can therefore be seen that accountability, as it applies to the NHS generally, is highly relevant to nursing.

This is clear from the so-called Heathrow Debate involving all of the Chief Nursing Officers for the United Kingdom (DoH 1993a). The participants saw that the general increase in accountability in the public services, particularly the health services, was going to have an impact on nursing. They also asked, in relation to strategic issues for the future of nursing, 'How will professional accountability, authority and responsibility be altered?' and this question was raised with specific reference to the community.

Accountability and professionalism

Owing to its dependence on such issues as authority and autonomy, the concept of accountability is closely related to the concept of professionalism. In 1992 I concluded that 'Accountability is the very essence of professionalism' (Watson 1992), with the justification that it sets professions apart from other kinds of occupations. However, it should be acknowledged that there are different ideas of what constitutes a profession. In most occupations the worker or practitioner is accountable to some extent for what they do. Not all of these occupations – and nursing could certainly be included – have complete authority over the work they do, and are therefore not fully autonomous. Nevertheless, the concept of accountability impinges on nurses generally in ways in which it does not impinge on many other non-professional occupations.

Nursing has some of the features of a profession in that training and a registered qualification are both required in order to practise (Thompson *et al.* 1994). By virtue of this nurses become accountable to the general public for their practice, and this accountability is regulated by a statutory body, the UKCC, which governs the training of nurses and holds the authority to remove individuals from the register and, thereby, their right to practise. This situation is analogous to other fields about whose professional status there is little doubt, such as medicine and the legal profession, in contrast to those who have a trade, for instance. Training and, possibly, listing by a governing body may be possible in certain trades. However, although individuals can be removed from a list they cannot actually be prevented from earning a living by means of that trade, in the way that nurses can be prevented from practising. In this light, therefore, the accountability of nurses lends nursing at least some of the features of a profession.

Accountable to whom?

As shown above, nurses are accountable to the public generally through their registration body, the UKCC. However, nurses, by virtue of the fact that they operate at the crossroads of many other professions, may have to be accountable in many other ways, in several directions and to a number of other bodies. These include the medical profession, health service management, individual patients and their families, and even educational institutions if they are seeking to update and improve their professional knowledge. Some of these directions require clarification.

The medical profession is, arguably, the one with which nurses work most closely. Nurses are increasingly taking on extended roles within their work and these usually involve some specialized training and subsequent examination in order to carry out the function autonomously. The most obvious example here is the administration of intravenous medication, but other everyday nursing procedures, such as the regular administration of prescribed medications, have their origins with the medical profession. As the authority to carry out such procedures does not at present lie with nurses, they cannot truly be said to be autonomous and, therefore must be held accountable to another, non-nursing, body.

The devolution of health service budgets down to unit level has brought nurses into an additional area of accountability which has increased their autonomy in the realm of spending at ward and unit level. However, the allocation of the budget is completely outwith the authority of nurses. Unit nursing managers may be the people to whom charge nurses are accountable for the operation of their budgets, but these will ultimately be accountable to non-nurses for the operation of the overall budget. There is a buffer-zone here in the accountability trail, as individual nurses would never be held to be accountable for their budgets to the ultimate body (the Department of Health or equivalent), but are exercising a level of accountability nevertheless.

Accountability to patients and relatives raises a further complication for nursing. Relatives may become involved in the accountability trail when individual patients are unable to make their own decisions, such as children, and adults who are mentally incompetent or unconscious. The complication arises because patients and their relatives comprise a particular part of the general population to whom nurses are already accountable through the UKCC. However, the relationship between nurses and patients introduces accountability in a very different way from the accountability which is exercised to a statutory body. Nurses may be expected to account for their actions and to explain procedures on a day-to-day basis, and this brings accountability very close to home. Nevertheless, such accountability is quite informal and a nurse is not obliged to be accountable, in the fullest sense, to patients and relatives. It has been argued, therefore, that nurses could be viewed as being accountable 'for' rather than 'to' individual patients and relatives (Watson 1992). Nurses are not unique in this and they share accountability of a kind, involving patients and relatives, with the medical profession. The situation for the medical profession, however, is very clear, certainly in legal terms. Doctors do not, for instance, have to take account of the wishes of relatives of incompetent adult patients, in arriving at a clinical decision to treat or not to treat (Watson 1994).

The complicated nature of accountability in nursing can, therefore, be seen from the above examples. At one extreme nurses are fully accountable to their statutory body. However, the number of occasions on which accountability to this body has to be 'made visible' are very few, and usually only arise in cases of misconduct. At the other extreme, nurses exercise daily and very visible accountability to bodies very close to them professionally and within the profession for aspects of nursing which are, ultimately, accounted for to bodies outside nursing.

The problem of multiple accountability

The question arises as to whether or not nurses are accountable to too many different bodies. Multiple accountability, as currently evidenced in universities, where research, audit procedures, teaching quality, research assessment and reporting to professional bodies all have to be operated by certain disciplines (including nursing departments in higher education establishments), has been questioned (Raman 1994). This raises a further dilemma for nursing: if professionalism is what we seek and accountability is one of the ways in which that professionalism will be either gained or conferred, then there must be an appropriate level of accountability, an optimum at which we can truly operate as a profession but at which the work for which we have trained and registered will not become stifled.

The process of achieving this optimum level of accountability will not be an easy one. There are multiple definitions of accountability and, even where some agreement exists, there is no real consensus on the extent of accountability that nurses currently operate. Furthermore, there are tensions both inside and outside the profession. Some see accountability as essential for certain types of nursing, and grasp the concept and its sequelae with enthusiasm. Although the climate may be such that hostile opposition to accountability is rarely voiced, there are certain situations (the use of eusol for wound cleansing being a perfect example) where nurses would gladly relinquish accountability in order to avoid the disputes which may arise with the medical profession (Tingle 1992a). Some outside the profession dismiss the whole concept and attempt to minimize nurses' potential fear of accountability by stating clearly that they are not really accountable for anything (Crossley 1993). Whatever direction the debate on accountability takes, it is surely self-evident that some resolution is in order.

This is an academic text and, as such, it does not set out to provide clear answers to the questions that surround accountability. Academics are unable to provide such answers, which lie with those in practice and with the professional and statutory bodies that govern nursing. Rather, this book sets out to illustrate the nature of accountability as it is operated in a variety of specialties, and illuminates this with the relevant philosophical, legal and ethical arguments. In addition, it sets out to inform the ongoing debate in and around the profession so that the matter of accountability can, perhaps, be seen more clearly, with its attendant difficulties, by a greater number of people.

HISTORICAL PERSPECTIVE

The development of nursing as an accountable profession, which is the title of Susan McGann's chapter, is inextricably linked with the historical development of the profession. According to McGann, accountability really began in 1919, with the passing of the Nurses' Registration Act. However, without the work of a number of key individuals at the end of the 19th century and the start of the 20th century, things might have been very different. A great many social and historical changes also played a part and it was, arguably, the mobilization of large numbers of women as nurses in the First World War which finally sealed the professional fate of nursing.

Florence Nightingale was a key figure in the professional development of nursing: indeed, she established the first formal training programmes for nurses. Nevertheless, it was never her intention that nurses should be registered, as she thought that this might mislead the public into accepting unsuitable women as nurses. She was concerned, in a much greater way, with the personal development and moral character of individual nurses. The movement to fully professionalize nursing was led by Mrs Bedford Fenwick, who was supported by her physician husband. However, there was still opposition within the profession to be overcome and one of the organizations, the Royal British Nurses Association, allowed doctors to become members. This body expelled Mrs Bedford Fenwick, and also voted against the registration of nurses.

It is probably more than coincidence that Florence Nightingale had died in 1910 and one of her allies in the battle against registration died in 1919, the very year when the first registration Act was passed by Parliament. The historical and political perspective offered by McGann certainly informs the present debate about accountability in nursing.

NURSING MODELS AND THE NURSING PROCESS

One of the ways in which nurses account for their work is by documentation. The nursing process, used within the framework of a model of nursing, is commonly the means by which documentation is structured. A text on accountability would therefore be incomplete without some consideration of nursing models and the nursing process. Helen Chalmers, in Chapter 3, describes the nursing process as a means whereby nurses account for their professional practice. Models are described as 'ways of thinking about nursing that highlight the need for particular kinds of knowledge and particular skills'.

Chalmers sees the grasping of accountability by nursing as a sign of professional maturity. This maturity also encompasses such concepts as teamwork and not feeling threatened by other groups of professionals. Many of the pressures which have led to the greater acceptance of accountability in nursing have come from outside the profession, in the shape of political decisions and structural changes in the health service. Nevertheless, accountability should be viewed positively.

Models of nursing have raised an awareness of the kind of knowledge which is required to practice. To quote Chalmers, nursing models take, as their starting point 'the nature of people' and, for example, using Orem's model of self-care, nurses are guided to view patients as people who are normally able and willing to undertake their own care but who, owing to a variety of circumstances, are unable to do so on occasion. A model such as Orem's will lead nurses to investigate the reasons why a person is unable to care for themselves and to acquire knowledge which will enable them to compensate or return them to self-care.

Models, by their nature, bring into question the very nature of nursing. Working within the conceptual framework of a model enables and obliges nurses to account for the things they do and, indeed, the things they do not do.

The nursing process, with its familiar four-step problem-solving approach to care, adds a further dimension in that it both requires and obliges nurses to document what they do. The act of documentation is one particular type of accountability which exposes individual nurses to scrutiny by their colleagues and by other professionals. The nursing process therefore encourages nurses to think clearly about what they are doing and to document it clearly, not only in order to be accountable for its own sake, but also that others may follow their thinking and provide a consistent pattern of care.

STANDARDS OF CARE

One of the ways in which nurses are increasingly being asked to account for the care they deliver is through the formulation and implementation of standards of care. A standard of care could almost be viewed as accounting in advance for what is going to be done; moreover, standards of care imply outcomes and audit, which are particular forms of accountability to which nurses are increasingly being exposed.

Lesley Duff explores the issues surrounding standards of care and accountability in her chapter. Through a discussion of relevant issues, such as disclosure and referent others, Duff explains how nursing is moving from largely external accountability to more internal accountability. Standards of care are one way in which this is being achieved. This has led nursing to derive clearer definitions of those things for which it has authority. Without this it is not possible to see clearly what nurses are responsible, and thereby accountable, for.

The difference between internal and external accountability is brought clearly into focus by Duff. She describes making a disclosure under a system of external accountability as 'recounting' rather than accounting. Clearly, the extent to which a nurse can be held accountable for a plan of action decided by someone else is limited. Nurses can only be held truly accountable for those things which they plan and execute themselves.

As already described, the implementation of standards of care is seen by Duff as being essential for the development of professional and personal accountability. Furthermore, underpinning the implementation of standards of care is the notion of research-based practice, and also educational issues whereby nurses become equipped to formulate their own standards and implement them in practice without necessarily having recourse to other professional groups. Of course, such developments are not without their drawbacks since, as nurses assume responsibility, accountability and making explicit their standards of care, they may become more liable to legal accountability for errors and omissions.

In the United Kingdom the Royal College of Nursing has been at the forefront in introducing standard setting and its counterpart, quality assurance, into nursing. This has not been done, however, without taking into account the different ways in which standards can be implemented and the potential conflicts that can arise. Viewed most superficially, one of the fundamental problems in standard setting is that, at some level, they can always be seen to have been imposed by someone else or some external body. This has consequences for accountability, since the greater the extent to which they have been imposed or are seen to be imposed, the less individuals will feel accountable for standards of care in their own clinical area. In order to overcome some of the potential conflicts, it is largely acknowledged that at least an element of the 'bottom up' approach is required in standard setting so that individuals and groups at the 'sharp end' of care delivery can feel that they own and are therefore accountable for those standards.

Quality assurance and the mechanism whereby it is carried out, namely audit, is not without its problems. As described by Duff, this can lead to conflict with other professional groups. Despite efforts to define areas of responsibility and accountability it is rarely the case, particularly in clinical work, that any one professional group is solely responsible for any aspect of care delivery. By implication, therefore, carrying out an audit of the activities of one group, such as nurses, will inevitably lead to the auditing of some aspects of the work of other groups, such as the medical profession. This could be overcome by mutually agreed standards, but this is not without its problems either.

Finally, Duff raises the question of whether or not standard setting and quality assurance are actually the best way of ensuring accountability in nursing. In particular, the position of the patient in all of this is discussed. Clearly, if nurses are in any way accountable to their patients then it is only proper that patients should be involved in the process of setting standards and measuring their implementation.

PRIMARY NURSING

Apart from the conceptual frameworks provided by nursing models, and regardless of how care is planned and documented, there are a number of ways in which nursing care can be delivered. All of these systems of care delivery can be viewed as being accountable, and thereby thrusting an element of accountability on to nurses, both individually and collectively. Traditional task allocation ensures that particular nurses are accountable for carrying out specific aspects of care for a large number of patients. This traditional approach has been modified into team nursing, whereby a team with an identified leader may be accountable either for a range of tasks or for a group of patients. However, the area where accountability is placed on the largest number of shoulders is, undoubtedly, primary nursing. It is only within this system of nursing that individual nurses – 'primary nurses' – are given responsibility, and thereby accountability, for the planning and delivery of care to specific patients from admission to discharge, and Sheila Rodgers discusses this in Chapter 5. The related issues of ability, responsibility and authority are also considered.

Accountability is not the only relevant issue: primary nursing, in contrast to task allocation or team nursing, requires a relatively large number of qualified and competent staff for its proper execution. Task allocation and team nursing can be carried out with relatively few qualified nurses, who oversee the work of others. In this light, therefore, primary nursing can be seen as expensive but having the potential to provide the highest quality of care. Rodgers examines team nursing and shows how closely related it is to task allocation, thereby lacking the essential elements of accountability which are seen in primary nursing. Primary nursing is also very much 'in vogue' in relation to current concepts such as the named nurse and other elements of what Rodgers describes as 'consumerism'.

Continuity of care is a key feature of primary nursing, the responsibility for which rests with the primary nurse, as opposed to the charge nurse in other care delivery systems. This leads, logically, to a discussion of the role of the charge nurse in primary nursing, and Rodgers explains how this is in no way diminished. Rather, it is crucial in that they are the people who must ensure that the ward is managed in such a way that primary nursing is facilitated. As such, not only are they responsible for implementing bureaucratic policies and playing their part in the line management of a hospital, but they must also ensure that the nurses in their charge are equipped both educationally and professionally for their roles as primary nurses.

Primary nursing raises further issues, such as relationships with medical staff, who may find it hard to change from the traditional approach of implementing decisions regarding individual patients via the charge nurse, and also the problems which may arise from what is, essentially, a system of devolved decision making at ward and unit level. Finally, although primary nursing undoubtedly increases the autonomy of individual nurses, Rodgers raises the question of whether or not it facilitates patient autonomy and whether it really leads to higher standards of care.

MIDWIFERY

Although Rosemary Mander acknowledges that most of the research and literature that was relevant to her chapter comes from nursing, this is somewhat surprising, as the concept of accountability is felt very strongly in midwifery and perhaps no other part of the profession is so acutely aware of the meaning and consequences of accountability. This is clearly exemplified in Mander's chapter.

Concentrating mainly on the individual accountability of the midwife rather than organizational accountability, Mander draws together many relevant strands of the literature. True accountability cannot exist without responsibility first being given – or taken – for particular areas of work. It has been the case, according to Etzioni (1975), that the term accountability has been misused and is often cynically applied to groups in order to win them over to particular points of view.

Mander traces the historical development of accountability in midwifery and looks at different aspects, such as institutional, personal and legislative accountability, and of course accountability to the mother. In contrast to nursing, it would appear that midwives may have actually lost responsibility – and, thereby, accountability – within their profession owing to the increasing medicalization of childbirth. The more ways in which obstetricians have taken responsibility for the 'abnormal' aspects of childbirth, particularly the diagnosis of problems, the more the role of the midwife has been reduced to that of 'obstetric nurse'; this is quite different, in Mander's estimation, from being a midwife.

Organizational changes in the provision of health services have likewise had a part to play in decreasing the responsibility of the midwife. Traditionally – and this was recognized in the Midwives Act of 1902 – midwives worked independently. However, in recent decades they have increasingly worked in hospitals. Mander discusses the reasons for this change, and it is interesting to juxtapose this with current trends towards home confinements.

The concepts of appropriate education and preparation, previously considered by both Rodgers and Chalmers in this volume, are relevant to the issue of accountability in midwifery. Without adequate preparation and academic training, midwives are unable to take on greater responsibility. It is Manders' view that in order to develop further, in terms of responsibility, autonomy and accountability, a substantial body of midwifery research needs to be established, separate from nursing and medical knowledge, and in this way midwives will be able to make full use of the regular refresher courses which they must attend in order to maintain the right to practise. The extension of accountability in midwifery will not be without its consequences, including litigation, and this is considered by Mander in the concluding section of her chapter.

PSYCHIATRIC NURSING

Stephen Tilley gives the issue of accountability within psychiatric nursing a very full treatment in his chapter. Not only does he see the issue of accountability as being as relevant in psychiatric nursing as in general nursing, he also sees it as being fundamental.

Altschul (1972), based on her earlier research, suggested that psychiatric nurses were not able to explain what they did in a way that made their practice accountable. Tilley, on the other hand, draws on his own research to show that there are forms of accountability made visible within psychiatric nursing. However, this is not necessarily expressed formally or even recognized as accountability. Tilley uses actual dialogue between psychiatric nurses and patients to demonstrate the accountability that is being exercised. The literature base of Tilley's work is both wide and deep. He draws on many sources within nursing research and also on the existentialist and postmodern writers to explain his observations.

THE COMMUNITY

One area where nurses work which raises accountability in a different way from most of the other areas considered in this volume is in the community. The community worker, be they district nurse, health visitor, community psychiatric nurse or midwife, tends to work alone. This raises its own challenges and problems.

Sarah Baggaley and Alison Bryans, in their chapter, look at community nursing mainly from the health visitor's perspective. They begin by defining the concept of community and then move on to consider recent and current government legislation which seeks to encourage a greater involvement of those in the community in health care. Further changes in the way health care is funded has meant that nurses working in the community are now providers of care who are purchased by general practitioners. This must have implications for the accountability of district nurses.

In common with other areas of nursing, the community sector is coming under increasing financial scrutiny – i.e. accountability in the monetary sense – and this has increased the pressure to alter the skill mix in favour of less qualified and non-qualified staff. Baggaley and Bryans see this as the opportunity which nurses in the community have to demonstrate the worth of what they do.

The issues of teamwork with others in the health team, and also how nursing work in the community relates to social care, have implications for the accountability of the nurse working in the community. One negative implication, according to Baggaley and Bryans, is that working alongside other groups and professionals may actually reduce the accountability of nurses towards individual patients.

Baggaley and Bryans, in common with many other authors in this volume, make the point that education and preparation for working in their particular area is essential in order for accountability to be properly exercised. This is particularly relevant to practice nurses who, in many cases, do not even have clear job descriptions; how can they be appropriately prepared?

Nurse prescribing may eventually affect all nurses, but it is liable to be most acutely relevant in the community. This adds another dimension to the accountability of the nurse. Perhaps it is analogous to the situations that prevail in the administration of intravenous medication by nurses.

Record keeping is fundamental to nursing. However, in the community it is essential because the patient is observed by the nurse only when visited and not, in a professional sense, in an ongoing way. It is necessary, therefore, to make clear records of visits and to assess the patient in such a way that meaningful comparisons can be made on future visits and by other members of the community team.

WORKING WITH CHILDREN

Paediatric nursing exposes a further aspect of accountability in nursing. Working with children entails the consent of responsible adults, and nurses must work with these adults in addition to those for whom they are caring. Gosia Brykczynska considers accountability in this highly specialized area of nursing, and also the philosophical underpinnings of paediatric nursing and accountability.

The scope of paediatric nursing has widened in recent years to include not only the ill or potentially ill child, but also the health and wellbeing of the child's family. Owing to the complex nature of paediatric nursing, involving many other professional groups as well as the family, accountability must be seen in the light of shared responsibility. Brykczynska considers what the specialized knowledge and responsibility of paediatric nursing consists of, and explains that it is wide ranging, from particular knowledge of the normal vital signs of a neonate to concern for wider social and political issues which have a bearing on the welfare of children.

Responsibility and accountability bring obligations and, according to Brykczynska, in the field of paediatric nursing there is an obligation to 'inculcate not only the requisite level of paediatric values that form the moral code of of paediatric nursing, but also the necessary amount of paediatric science and care'.

Shared accountability with parents is a particularly interesting area for paediatric nursing. This is due to the fact that consent is normally required for surgical procedures to be carried out on children. Brykczynska makes the point that the surgeon may know what the appropriate procedure is for a child but that the parents have to be helped in their decision – i.e. to be accountable – to permit the procedure. Paediatric nurses have a key role to play here. Conversely, they also have a role when parents decide not to proceed with an investigation or operation.

Children with chronic illness involve the paediatric nurse in helping such children to take responsibility for their own treatment; for example, instructing diabetic children to administer their own insulin necessitates handing over responsibility, and therefore accountability, to those children. Once responsibility has been handed over it cannot easily or reasonably be taken back, and this raises its own particular problems. Brykczynska concludes with an interesting philosophical consideration of the issues related to authority and accountability and how these impinge on children, parents, society and paediatric nurses.

LEGAL ACCOUNTABILITY

There are circumstances under which nurses may be held legally accountable for what they do. This accountability, which can have severe penalties beyond dismissal and removal from the professional register, must be seen in its own light, and John Tingle investigates this in Chapter 10. The concept of negligence, whereby an individual nurse may be held responsible for an action or omission, is described as vicarious liability and may lead to the nurse's employer also being held legally accountable for such negligence.

Where negligence or vicarious liability has been established, Tingle describes what the aim of the law is in dealing with such matters. This encompasses a great many features, including deterrence and compensation. However, the nurse is not only legally accountable but also accountable in a great many other ways, all of which may require separate explanations, or accounts, of actions. A variety of sanctions can be imposed but the severest, those of imprisonment and payment of compensation, lie with the law.

Some interesting studies are presented by Tingle and many of these are taken from published legal cases. The potential conflicts faced by nurses, for example when working in poorly resourced areas but still attempting to do the best they can and failing to provide a high standard of care or committing an error, are covered. Using mainly medical examples from published legal cases, Tingle shows how the law attempts to deal with cases of individual and collective professional misconduct. On the whole, the judges and courts seem to act reasonably and demonstrate a remarkable understanding of the difficulties faced by busy dedicated professionals, while at the same time attempting to safeguard the health and safety of the public.

ETHICS AND ACCOUNTABILITY

In at least one language – Spanish – there is no equivalent word for accountability. Kath Melia uses this to make the point that the relationship between ethics and accountability is not entirely clear, as accountability is simply about lines of responsibility and not values. On the other hand, the ethical dimension to responsibility – one of the components of accountability – is undeniable, and it is only in this respect that there may be an ethical component to accountability.

LIFE AND DEATH DECISIONS

It is hard to imagine an area of caring where the issue of accountability comes into focus more and carries greater consequences than in decisions about life and death. Hazel McHaffie covers this area extensively in her chapter, and in doing so raises a great many pertinent issues. There has been no shortage of contemporary cases in the United Kingdom concerning the issues of life and death, particularly with regard to decisions about whether or not to continue treatment, or to administer lethal treatment where the outcome will be certain death. The Tony Bland and Dr Cox cases come to mind (see below), and these are both used as examples by McHaffie.

It is undoubtedly the case that nurses have not traditionally been at the forefront in matters of life and death decision making. However, McHaffie makes the point that 'it is entirely inappropriate for them to abdicate responsibility' in these matters. With reference to the cases mentioned above, for example, nurses had to continue to administer care to the dying Tony Bland after the decision was taken to withdraw hydration, and it was a nurse who drew attention to the fact that a lethal injection had been administered to an elderly patient, albeit at that patient's request, by Dr Cox.

The complexity of accountability is well illustrated by these cases. Dr Cox acted, without recourse to discussion with any external bodies, out of a sense of accountability to his patient who, with the support of her family, had requested an end to her suffering. Sister Hart, who reported him, acted according to the letter of her professional code of conduct, and thereby exercised her accountability to that professional body. Dr Howe, who was the consultant responsible for Tony Bland, turned to the courts for a decision on terminating active treatment for his patient, despite the support of Tony Bland's family. McHaffie returns to these cases several times in order to illustrate points in her chapter.

The issue of euthanasia per se is extremely complex at the sharp end of health-care delivery. The word itself has been misconstrued and can mean almost anything the user wants it to mean. Literally translated, euthanasia simply means a 'good death', and this is something all health-care professionals would wish for those in their care. In British law it is clearly wrong to deliberately hasten someone's death by any means. This leaves plenty of scope for the administration of drugs which, while they may also hasten death, are given primarily to ease suffering. Extraordinary means of life support can be withdrawn if it can be shown that a person is, essentially, dead. Nevertheless, there are numerous grey areas in medicine where the above cases do not entirely fit, and although medical staff are ultimately responsible for making and implementing any decisions about the withdrawal of treatment, the accountability of the whole team, including nurses, is called into question in the process. This new attitude towards accountability, whereby the input of the nursing profession is acknowledged, is exemplified by the combined Royal College of Nursing and British Medical Association document on resuscitation (BMA and RCN 1993).

McHaffie illustrates many of the examples to which she refers with pertinent case studies which are directly relevant to nursing. One point she makes is the fact that the decision to withdraw treatment does *not* entail a withdrawal of care. That care, moreover, may extend to many significant people other than the dying patient. However, this can lead to problems. What happens, for instance, to the nurse who does not agree, either for personal moral reasons or for reasons specifically related to a case, with a decisions not to treat?

Obviously there are no easy answers, but the necessity for teamwork in arriving at such decisions is highlighted as at least one way of arriving at and implementing correct decisions.

RESEARCH

This volume is probably uniquely privileged in having the first thorough consideration of the accountability of the nursing researcher. Alison Tierney begins with the idea that research is a prime responsibility of an accountable profession, and in so doing echoes the sentiments regarding preparation of the profession, both individually and collectively, which are expressed in some of the other chapters. The Department of Health in the United Kingdom has recently considered the issue of research in nursing and in the health service generally (DoH 1993b). It is clear that nursing research has much to contribute towards both the development of the profession and the provision of health services.

In common with other areas of accountability in nursing, accountability in nursing research is, at least, a dual notion. As Tierney explains, nurses as researchers are accountable per se in all of the ways in which other researchers are accountable. However, nurses in research are also accountable as nurses for the ethical and caring conduct of their research. In this light the UKCC *Code of Professional Conduct* (UKCC 1992a) applies to nurses in research every bit as much as it applies to other nurses. Researchers generally are also accountable in a number of other ways, all of which apply to nurses. For example, researchers are accountable to funding bodies and to the public generally. Research has to be carried out as specified in research proposals, and the outcome of the research must be presented in the form of accounts. These accounts are usually aimed at the funding body and at the public through research publications. The latter are usually refereed, an account thereby being given anonymously to an unknown person or persons. A further aspect of accountability in nursing research, in common with medical research and other forms of research involving human subjects, is to ethical committees. Such accounts, in common with proposals, have to be given in advance of the research being carried out. Any deviation from the proposed research, particularly involving undesirable outcomes to participants, may have to be accounted for. In the case of a nurse an account would have to be given to their statutory body and even to a court of law. Such accountability is amply covered by Tingle in his chapter.

Nevertheless, despite these multiple forms of accountability, research nurses essentially work in isolation from any overseeing body. In this way, therefore, they are morally accountable and this is often only to themselves. They are morally accountable for carrying out the research in the way they have proposed, and in gathering data and subsequently publishing in a way that does not misrepresent what they have done. Deviation from such moral accountability may or may not be detected. If it is detected then the prospect of obtaining further funding or ethical permission for research is severely reduced.

Accountability to participants in research must also be exercised, and partly in advance of the research itself. Usually some kind of consent will be required if human subjects are to be involved and, in order for this to be obtained, an accurate account of what being involved in the research will mean to the participant will have to be given. Thereafter, the researcher is accountable to participants for conducting the research in the way that has been specified. Tierney considers some of the ways in which researchers are accountable to participants, including the exercising of confidentiality.

NURSING EDUCATION

At several points throughout this volume the issue of nursing education as a means of instilling the appropriate training, knowledge and attitudes in nurses has been raised. It is only right, therefore, that the issue of accountability in nursing education should be addressed and, as will be seen from Diane Marks-Maran's chapter, this presents something of a moving target, owing to the many changes which have taken place in this decade in the structures of nursing, health boards and, as a result, nursing education.

Nurse education, surely, has always been accountable to those it educates and also to those who receive health care from nurses. Recently, however, with the introduction of the purchaser–provider concept into health care, nurse education is finding itself accountable to health boards and trusts, and also to institutes of higher education, which are increasingly absorbing the former colleges of nursing. This new era has implications for the planning and delivery of nursing education. There is an immediate conflict for colleges of nursing between achievement-led education, which has as its object the development of individuals, and the outcome-based approach inherent in the purchaser–provider split, which is concerned merely with the products of nursing education. Nursing education cannot abandon the former without doing a disservice to its students, but must take into account the latter or it will not be funded by health trusts.

The issue of multiple accountability, raised at the beginning of this chapter, is of course directly relevant to nursing education. As nursing education enters higher, university-based education institutions it will become open to scrutiny by a host of additional bodies, both within and outwith the institution. The existing departments of nursing in universities have had to account to their respective national boards for their courses so that they can be accredited for registration of their students on the new (Project 2000) parts of the professional register. At the same time, they are having to account to their academic funding bodies for such things as research assessment, academic audit and teaching quality assessment. Any hope that colleges of nursing had of avoiding such scrutiny will have been dashed by the government's proposals to move all of nursing education into the higher education/university sector. Marks-Maran identifies this as 'biculturalism', but it is doubtful whether this is sufficient to describe the multifaceted kinds of accountability that nursing education will have to operate in the near future.

CONCLUSION

The issue of accountability in nursing is complex and multifaceted. Generally, it is viewed positively and has been adopted with enthusiasm. This volume gives the subject comprehensive consideration by a number of selected authors, many of whom are recognized experts in their field. Historically, nurses strove to become a profession, an accountable and self-regulating body. In the more recent past, the pressures on the profession in the direction of greater accountability have been largely externally driven by other professional groups, and by changes in the structure and funding of the health services in the United Kingdom. For the future, it can only be hoped that the issue is adopted, analysed and shaped by those in the profession. To do otherwise will be allowing others to define the boundaries and the details of professional nursing practice.

2 | The development of nursing as an accountable profession

Susan McGann

INTRODUCTION

The modern concept of professional accountability, applied to nursing, assumes that the nurse is a member of a profession. It depends on individual nurses being aware of their membership of a profession and accepting that status, with the rights and responsibilities that go with it (White 1977). With the passing of the Nurses Registration Acts, in 1919, nurses in Britain achieved the status of an accountable profession. This meant that registered nurses were legally accountable for their work and could be struck off the register for unprofessional behaviour. However, the concept of professional accountability is more intangible than legal accountability. In order for it to flourish, nurses had to become strong in their own professional self-esteem. This did not happen after 1919. Before considering why, we must look at the development of professional awareness among nurses.

HISTORICAL PERSPECTIVE

The year 1887 was the turning point in the emergence of nursing as a profession. In this year, the first professional organization for nurses was founded, the British Nurses' Association (BNA), and this marked the point when British nurses set their sights on professional status. It was inevitable that, sooner or later, efforts would be made to standardize the training of nurses and professional consciousness would emerge, but it took another 30 years before the majority of nurses in Britain realized the need for a professional organization.

Once nurses had joined a professional association in large numbers, they achieved state registration. The years between 1887 and 1919 were a period of professionalization for nurses everywhere, which reflected the growth of the women's movement in America and the suffrage campaign in Britain (Benson 1990).

By the end of the 19th century, hospitals were no longer seen as charitable institutions for the sick poor but places where scientific medicine and surgery were practised, and they began to attract more patients, including the middle classes. The corresponding growth in the number of hospital beds depended on an increasing number of nurses to work in the hospitals. There was also an expansion of the nurse's duties as the 'trained' nurse evolved in response to the advances in medicine. Nurses at the end of the 19th century were performing tasks – such as taking temperatures – which 20 years earlier no doctor would have delegated to them (Morten 1895). These two related factors, the advances in medicine and the expansion in the number of hospital beds, produced a sharp rise in the number of nurse training schools in the country (Baly 1986).

The matrons of the time were aware of the rapid changes that were taking place in nursing and the uncontrolled nature of the development (Fenwick 1897; Stewart 1905). By 1886 the development of nursing was such that the Hospitals Association (HA) appointed a committee to consider the possibility of establishing a register of nurses. Against the advice of the nurse members, the committee decided to set the standard for a registered nurse at 1 year's training. The matrons resigned from the Association and founded the BNA in 1887, the first professional association for nurses.

THE BRITISH NURSES' ASSOCIATION

The founders of the BNA were predominantly educated, middle-class women who had entered nursing in the 1860s and 1870s, under the inspiration of Florence Nightingale's work (McGann 1992). They had received little in the way of formal training and, having risen to the top of the nursing world, as matrons of large teaching hospitals, they were imbued with the spirit of pioneers. They had seen nurses develop from being the 'handywoman' of the 1860s and 1870s into the trained nurse with 3 years' systematic training in a hospital, able to share in the intellectual side of medicine. They saw nursing as an opportunity to improve society and as an area where an intelligent woman could make a career for herself. They had no doubt that the work of nurses was of such importance to the community that it required a system of registration. This would protect the public from the untrained nurse and it would protect the trained nurse from the competition of untrained women.

Mrs Bedford Fenwick

This group of matrons, who became the leaders of the movement to profession-alize nursing, was led by Mrs Bedford Fenwick, a former matron of St Bartholomew's Hospital, and Isla Stewart, her successor there. Following the example of the medical profession, which was their natural role model and which had achieved state registration in 1858, they set out to achieve state regis-tration for nurses. They were determined to set the standard for registration as high as the best nurses, in other words, 3 years' training, and believed that the only way to achieve this was by establishing a statutory system of registration, since a voluntary system would never reach the poorer hospitals. Mrs Fenwick outlined the requirements of a Nurses' Registration Act to the first meeting of the BNA. The Act would set up a General Nursing Council (GNC), which would be a legally recognized body. This Council, composed largely of the heads of the nursing profession, would be responsible for setting the standard of training, examination and registration (Fenwick 1887).

The leaders of the campaign for state registration realised that one of the keys to professional status was the education of nurses. Owing to the rapid evolution of nurses' training schools, the majority were schools only in name (Fenwick 1897). Each hospital had developed its own system of training in isolation. Standards varied greatly, from the big teaching hospitals at one end of the scale to the small cottage hospitals at the other end. As a result of this 'free for all', the term 'trained' nurse could mean anything. The progressives regarded the introduction of a uniform system of training, followed by a standard examina-tion, as a priority (Stewart 1895). They wanted to remove the uncertainty and ambiguity of the position of the trained nurse: 'We are fully determined that, in the future, the public shall know as precisely what is meant by a trained nurse as what is meant by a qualified medical man, and the nurse's right to her title, free from the intrusion of unqualified women, shall be as unquestioned as his' (Mollett 1898).

Mrs Fenwick enumerated the profession's most pressing needs in her speech to the International Council of Nurses' Congress in 1901: preliminary education before entering the hospital wards; postgraduate teaching to keep abreast of developments; instruction as nurse teachers; a state-constituted board to exam-ine and maintain discipline; and legal status to protect their professional rights and to ensure professional autonomy. She saw the choice facing nurses clearly:

'We stand now at the Rubicon...we must either go forward or go back...before us lies the organized and scientific profession of our dreams, in which every duly qualified nurse is registered as a skilled practitioner. Behind us is that dreary downhill path, descending to a disorganized vocation of obsolete methods, in the ranks of which all kinds and condi-tions of workers, good, bad and indifferent, struggle and compete' (Fenwick 1901a).

The campaign for the state registration of nurses divided the hospital and nursing world into two camps. Those who were in favour of professional autonomy for nurses supported the campaign; those who did not want to see nursing become a profession opposed it. The opposition numbered among its members many influential persons from the medical and hospital establishment and, from the nursing establishment itself, no less a figure than Florence Nightingale. Miss Nightingale was opposed to any system of public registration for nurses (Stewart 1895; Cook 1913). She considered that it could only mislead the public into thinking that a registered nurse was a good nurse, whereas the qualities of a good nurse were just those qualities which could never be judged by a theoretical examination. She opposed all attempts to professionalize nursing, believing that nursing was a vocation and an art, and should only be followed by those who had a 'calling' (Cook 1913).

Eva Luckes, the Matron of the London Hospital, shared Miss Nightingale's views about nursing and the two women became friends through their shared opposition to state registration. Miss Luckes regretted the growing tendency among nurses and the public to overrate both the importance and the amount of technical knowledge that a nurse should possess. She believed the human side of a nurse's work would always be more important: 'People too frequently forget that nursing is an Art...nursing must not be regarded merely as a profession' (Luckes 1914).

PROFESSIONAL REGISTRATION

In 1892 the British Nurses' Association, which had been granted the prefix 'Royal' (RBNA), announced its intention to apply for a royal charter authorizing it to form a register of trained nurses. The opponents of registration feared that this would give the RBNA undue influence over nurses. The issue became one of intense public debate, with both sides lobbying in support of their case. In the end, the Privy Council steered a middle course. The charter was granted but it did not empower the RBNA to set up a register of trained nurses who could call themselves 'registered' or 'chartered'. Instead, it could maintain 'a list of persons who may have applied to have their names entered therein as nurses' (Cook 1913).

Matrons' Council of Great Britain and Ireland

Following this success, the opponents of registration gained control of the RBNA. Membership was also open to doctors, and when the Association was founded many eminent physicians and surgeons had been invited to join. Under the terms of the new charter, they were able to gain control and remove Mrs Fenwick from the Council. Two years later, they succeeded in carrying a vote against registration.

This experience was not wasted on nursing leaders, as it brought home to them the strength of feeling of the opposition to state registration for nurses. They realized that any attempt to promote the status of nursing would arouse 'prehistoric prejudices' and 'a multitude of vested interests' (Dock 1899, 1901). At the International Council of Nurses' Congress, in 1901, Catherine Wood, former Lady Superintendent of Great Ormond Street Hospital and one of the founders of the RBNA, spoke of the lessons they had learnt:

> 'In England we have tried the experiment of organizing the profession in conjunction with the medical profession, but with disastrous results; it is a failure...we must be free to organize ourselves; the relation of man to woman complicates the situation; the relative position of doctor and nurse makes it impossible. Though our work is in common, the details differ, and though we do not claim independence of the medical profession, we claim freedom to discuss our own affairs, to make our own laws, to decide on common principles of work' (Wood 1901).

After her expulsion from the RBNA Mrs Fenwick, and Miss Stewart, who had resigned from the Association, founded the Matrons' Council of Great Britain and Ireland. Membership was restricted to matrons and superintendents of nurses, and the aim was to provide members with a forum for discussing professional issues. They were all agreed that the priority for the profession was a uniform system of training and state registration (Stewart 1898). A strong influence on Mrs Fenwick at this time was the American women's movement. In 1892 she travelled to Chicago to organize the British nursing section at the World's Fair, to be held there in 1893. This was very successful, but the most lasting effect of her trips to Chicago was her contact with Mrs May Wright Sewall, founder of the International Council of Women, and her friendship with Isabel Hampton Robb, the director of the Nursing Department at the John Hopkins Hospital in Baltimore, and her assistant Lavinia Dock. These two women, Robb and Dock, were leading the move to professionalize nurses in the United States (James 1979).

Miss Robb and Mrs Fenwick seized the opportunity presented by the inclusion, for the first time, of a Women's Section at the World's Fair, to publicize the new profession of nursing. They planned a conference on nursing, for which Miss Robb carefully chose a series of papers that illustrated the developments in nursing and the need for a higher standard of education. At the conference, Miss Robb spoke of the responsibility of hospitals to provide nurses with a real education in return for the nursing services rendered. She believed that the pioneer generation of schools was no longer good enough (James 1979).

When she returned from Chicago, Mrs Fenwick became involved in the organization of the 1899 Congress of the International Congress of Women, to be held in London. Once again she took the opportunity to organize a nursing section, which attracted a considerable number of foreign nurses. These delegates were invited to attend the annual meeting of the Matrons' Council, held the day after the Congress (McGann 1992). The guest speaker at this meeting was Mrs May Wright Sewall, the President of the International Council of Women, who addressed the meeting on the subject of professional organization:

'One of the chief objects of organization is to get professional recognition, to command the respect from the public which you think you deserve. As an isolated individual you are unable to do it...when you come into your peerage you can establish laws which will govern your wages, and that will put you into a different attitude toward the public and the public will pay to each individual the respect it pays to the organization' (Sewall 1905).

At this meeting Mrs Fenwick proposed the establishment of an International Council of Nurses (ICN), which would be organized on the same basis as the International Council of Women, membership being based on one national association to represent the nurses of each country. The ICN, which came into existence the following year, strengthened the efforts of nurses for professional improvement in all countries. It organized international congresses, which encouraged nurses to discuss questions of common interest and importance to their profession (Fenwick 1901b). The leaders of the campaign to professionalize nursing valued these contacts with nurses in other countries. Mrs Fenwick's journal, The Nursing Record and Hospital World, renamed The British Journal of Nursing in 1902, became the official organ of the ICN and carried her ideas on the professional status of nurses around the world.

The Matrons' Council was concerned about the need to raise professional awareness among nurses in Britain. In the United States nurses had followed the example of university graduates and started to form alumnae associations. The first had been formed in 1891, and by 1897 the majority of training schools in America and Canada had them. These associations provided the nurses with a professional organization which could look after their social, economic, educational and professional interests. Following a paper by Miss Robb on the subject, to the Matrons' Council, Miss Stewart proposed the formation of the League of St Bartholomew's Nurses. The League, the first of its kind in this country, was inaugurated in December 1899 (McGann 1992). Over the next 10 years five more Leagues were formed, based on training schools, and in 1904 a National Council of Nurses was set up, composed of delegates from the existing nurses' societies and associations, to represent British nurses in the International Council of Nurses.

POLITICAL PERSPECTIVE

The process of professionalization of nurses continued in the years leading up to the First World War. At an international level, the ICN held meetings and congresses in Berlin in 1904, in Paris in 1907, in London in 1909, and in

Cologne in 1912. For nurses campaigning for professional status and registration, against prejudice and apathy in their own countries, the international meetings were of the greatest value: 'It is an inspiration and source of encouragement to know that other countries are facing the same problems, working towards the same common standards' (Robb 1909).

In the early years of this century, the campaigners had reason to be optimistic about achieving state registration. In 1902 a Midwives Act was passed, establishing a Central Midwives Board and introducing the registration of midwives in England. In 1905, a Select Committee of the House of Commons reported in favour of state registration for nurses, and the following year the British Medical Association (BMA) voted almost unanimously in favour of state registration for nurses. Nurses were achieving legal status in other countries, first in South Africa in 1891, when the Cape Medical Council took on the responsibility for registering trained nurses; in Natal in 1899; then in New Zealand in 1901; in four states in the United States in 1903; and in the Transvaal in 1906. By 1914 40 of the American States and the Scandinavian countries had state registration of nurses (BJN 1903; Nursing Times 1921).

Early registration bill

In Britain, the first bill for the registration of nurses was introduced to parliament in 1904 as a Private Member's bill. It had been drawn up by Mrs Fenwick and Miss Stewart, with the assistance of Dr Bedford Fenwick, who fully supported his wife's campaign for the professional status of nurses. They had formed the Society for the State Registration of Nurses in 1902 to lead the campaign for registration. A second Private Member's bill for the registration of nurses was introduced in parliament in 1904 on behalf of the RBNA. Although it was now promoting a bill for the registration of nurses, it was, in Mrs Fenwick's words, an employers' bill, giving the controlling vote on the proposed GNC to hospital and medical authorities. The bill drafted by the Fenwicks gave a majority of the seats on the proposed council to nurses, thus ensuring that nurses had professional autonomy.

It was at this point that the Select Committee of the House of Commons was appointed to inquire into the subject. The Committee heard evidence from witnesses representing the medical and nursing professions, and from lay people, including Dr and Mrs Bedford Fenwick, Isla Stewart and Miss Luckes. The Committee reported in favour of state registration and accepted that 3 years was the most practical period for the training of a nurse. The pro-registration party were confident that statutory recognition of their profession could no longer be postponed, but they slowly realized that the government had no plans to draw up a nurses' registration bill and, when the two Private Members' bills for registration were reintroduced in the House of Commons, they were defeated.

A third bill for registration was promoted in 1908, this time in the House of Lords. This bill proposed an 'official directory' of nurses, instead of a legal system of registration, and was promoted by the opponents of professional autonomy for nurses. The bill made no provision for a minimum standard of training or for a GNC. Mrs Fenwick described it as 'the Nurses' Enslavement Bill', and its defeat was interpreted as a sign of support for the cause of state registration. The Fenwicks' bill was then introduced in the Lords and was passed but, once again, without government support, it failed to get a reading in the Commons.

A feeling of frustration set in among the leaders of the campaign for registration in 1909, after a delegation to the Prime Minister had failed to obtain any guarantee of support for registration. It was decided to form a Central Committee for the State Registration of Nurses, which would represent the eight existing associations of trained nurses in the country, to promote a joint bill. The bill incorporated the three principles which Mrs Fenwick regarded as beyond compromise: a minimum standard of 3 years' training as the qualification for registration; a uniform curriculum and examination for all nurses; and the appointment of a general nursing council to be responsible for professional standards.

This joint bill was introduced in the House of Commons, as a Private Members' bill, in 1910, and each year after that up to 1914, but failed to get a hearing. Miss Dock remarked: 'There are those who believe that no woman's bill will seem important to the House of Commons until women are fully enfranchised' (Dock 1912). Mrs Fenwick shared this view: as a suffragist for many years she believed that the nurses' campaign for legal recognition was part of women's struggle for the right to professional status and autonomy. This view was given weight by the fact that the opposition was not against registration in itself: it had in fact proposed several systems of registration over the years, but would oppose any system of registration that gave nurses legal status and professional autonomy.

The government argued that they could not afford to ignore the opponents of registration, and there is no doubt that the opponents commanded real influence. But, as Miss Stewart said in 1905, the real enemies of registration were the rank and file of nurses, numbering ostensibly 70 or 80 000, who through their apathy allowed the government to do nothing (Stewart 1905). The number of nurses who supported state registration through membership of one of the nurses' organizations, estimated at 10 000, was a small minority of the total number of nurses in the country. When the First World War started in 1914, the Central Committee's bill for state registration had just received a majority at its first reading in the House of Commons, but had been refused a second reading. With the outbreak of war, the facility to promote Private Members' bills was suspended.

THE WAR

The war saw the mobilization of thousands of nurses. Over 10 000 joined the regular army nursing service, Queen Alexandra's Imperial Military Nursing Service, and saw action at the front (Haldane 1923). Through the Territorial Army Nursing Service approximately 6000 nurses were employed in the temporary military hospitals at home and abroad (McGann 1992). Another 6000 nurses were deployed, through the British Red Cross Society (BRCS), in the auxiliary hospitals at home and abroad. Finally, there were over 12 000 VADs, the untrained women who worked as nurses through the Voluntary Aid Detachments run by the BRCS.

At the start of the war the government had delegated responsibility for the organization of the voluntary medical and nursing services to the BRCS. The nursing profession was dismayed that after 20 years of campaigning for the professional status of trained nurses, the government still regarded nursing as philanthropic work. In the first 5 months of the war, from August to December of 1914, many auxiliary hospitals were set up by wealthy ladies with no nursing experience. The National Council of Trained Nurses placed on record its disapproval of the nursing of sick and wounded soldiers in military and auxiliary hospitals by 'untrained and unskilled women' (BJN 1915a). This was an attack on the VADs and the amateur hospitals which had been encouraged by the BRCS.

By the beginning of 1915, the unorganized state of nursing was beginning to cause problems. The government found it necessary to tighten up the issue of passports to nurses going to work abroad. It had been found that many women volunteering for nursing work abroad were untrained, and on arrival at their destination were an embarrassment to the authorities. Sarah Swift, as the Matron-in-Chief of the BRCS, had the job of checking the qualifications of all the nurses volunteering for work at home and abroad. In 1915 she also became responsible for interviewing and selecting VADs who volunteered for nursing (McGann 1992).

The nursing profession had advised from the start that these untrained women should only be allowed to nurse in the auxiliary hospitals, and then under the supervision of trained nurses. By the spring of 1915 there was such a shortage of nurses that it became necessary to allow the VADs to work in the wards of military hospitals, albeit again under supervision. Mrs Fenwick pointed out that, had registration been introduced before the war, the shortage of nurses would have been foreseen and a register of nurses would have been available to check their qualifications and to provide a means of communicating with trained nurses (BJN 1915b).

By the end of 1915, Miss Swift had come to the conclusion that the unorganized state of nursing was 'chaos', and in no-one's interest, least of all nurses'. She felt that to wait until after the war for a system of state registration would be too late, as by that time thousands of VADs would be competing with trained nurses. She thought the profession should organize itself on a voluntary basis. She proposed the establishment of a College of Nursing, to be run by nurses with the cooperation of the training schools. The College would introduce a uniform curriculum of training and recognize approved training schools, grant certificates and maintain a register of nurses who had received these certificates.

She enlisted the support of Arthur Stanley, the Chairman of the BRCS and, as Treasurer of St Thomas' Hospital, an influential person among hospital governors, and three eminent matrons, Alicia Lloyd Still, Matron of St Thomas' Hospital, Rachel Cox-Davies, Matron of the Royal Free Hospital, and Miss Haughton, Matron of Guy's Hospital. They wrote to the matrons and managers of the large teaching hospitals around the country proposing the scheme for a College of Nursing and asking for their support. After 3 months of discussions the College was launched in April 1916, with the support of the training schools (McGann 1992).

The old state registration party was opposed to the College of Nursing. They believed that it was only a matter of time before the government accepted the necessity for state registration and they were not prepared to accept a voluntary system. Mrs Fenwick in particular would not countenance the involvement of hospital managers in the professional affairs of nurses. Her vision for many years had been of an independent nursing profession, governed by an independent general nursing council. Prolonged negotiations between the promoters of the College and the state registration party took place. They all recognized that conditions had changed since before the war, and that the time was right for a new initiative. Many of the old campaigners were won over when the founders of the College agreed to make a bill for state registration a priority.

The membership of the College of Nursing grew rapidly, despite the fact that the war was still going on and nurses were scattered all over the country and abroad. By the end of 1916 there were 2000 members; by the end of 1917 the number was 8000, and by 1919 it had reached 13 000. The rank and file of nurses were joining a professional organization for the first time. The Council of the College attempted to reach agreement with the Central Committee for the State Registration of Nurses over a joint bill. Negotiations finally broke down in 1918, and the two groups promoted separate bills, the Central Committee's in the House of Commons and the College's in the Lords.

REGISTRATION ACT 1919

A majority of the profession was now agreed on the need for registration and the government appears to have accepted registration in principle at this point (Abel-Smith 1960). The Minister of Health, Dr Addison, negotiated with the College and the Central Committee in an attempt to reach an agreed bill, but when this proved impossible he asked the two parties to withdraw their bills and promised a government bill. This was introduced in parliament in November

1919, and became law in December. Separate Acts for Scotland and Ireland were passed. After a campaign of over 30 years, nurses in Britain had achieved the status of an accountable profession.

There are several reasons why the government was prepared to give nurses state registration in 1919 and not before: the opposition from within the profession had disappeared; Florence Nightingale had died in 1910; and Miss Luckes died in February 1919. Nurses were becoming more politicized: 20 000 had joined the College of Nursing between 1916 and 1920. The opposition from the medical profession and hospital governors had been won over by giving them a consultative role in the College of Nursing.

In the wider world of politics the issue, like women's suffrage, was no longer a football for party politics, which it had been before the war. The status of women had benefited from their war work and the principle of female suffrage had been accepted when women over 30 were given the vote in 1918. Some Members of Parliament feared the growing industrial unrest would spread to women workers. During the war the number of women joining trade unions had increased sharply. There was also the threat that if state registration was withheld any longer, nurses would be driven into the arms of the Labour Party, who had made an issue of their poor wages and conditions (Dingwall *et al.* 1988).

CONCLUSIONS

Like the achievement of women's suffrage, registration did not prove to be the turning point in the profession's progress (Carter 1939). The 'battle of the nurses' for and against registration, had ended in the compromise of the 1919 Nurses Registration Acts. Unlike the Midwives Act of 1902, the Nurses Registration Acts did not give nurses legal status, and nursing by unregistered women calling themselves nurses was not prohibited. This created a second grade of nurse outside the control of the three General Nursing Councils. In addition to the register of general nurses, the Acts established supplementary registers for male nurses, mental nurses, nurses of 'mental defectives', sick childrens' nurses and fever nurses. This was professionally divisive, and prevented the development of a comprehensive general training scheme.

Mrs Fenwick believed at first that, having won a two-thirds majority of nurses on the GNC, they had secured professional autonomy. However, her vision of a nursing profession equal in status to the medical profession was not to be. The government had designed that the Act was 'confined within the smallest possible compass' (Dingwall *et al.* 1988), and all the decisions of the GNC were subject to the approval of the Minister of Health and of both Houses of Parliament. The first intervention came from parliament when the rules drawn up by the Council for the registration of existing nurses were significantly altered by the Commons. The definition of 'existing nurse' was widened to include a level of experienced but untrained nurses that the majority of the profession considered unwise. When the Council drafted a syllabus of training, based on the syllabus in use at the Nightingale School at St Thomas' Hospital, the Minister refused to make it compulsory. He considered that it demanded too high a standard of general education from probationers and was impractical for training schools. The syllabus remained advisory. Again, on the inspection of training schools the Minister refused to ratify the scheme drawn up by the Council and, without any financial provision for inspectors, members of the Council had to carry out limited inspections themselves (McGann 1992). There was nothing in the Act to prohibit training schools which had not been approved by the Council, training nurses.

The power of the profession, through the General Nursing Councils, to raise professional standards was very limited. The educational standards the nurse leaders had set out to achieve through state registration were diluted or obstructed by both the government and parliament. Any attempt by the Councils to improve the standard of training was weighed against the cost implications for the hospitals. By 1920 the hospitals had become totally dependent on the provision of cheap nursing services provided by the nurse training schools. The hospitals were running on deficit budgets by this time, and a threat to the supply of nursing recruits would make matters worse. The apprenticeship system of training, evolved to deal with the conditions in the 19th-century hospitals, was out of date, but hospital economics depended on its survival (Baly 1986). This system of training, with its emphasis on discipline and conformity, produced nurses who were obedient and uncritical (Helmstadter 1993). On top of this, the hierarchical organization of nursing in hospitals produced a hierarchy of accountability, which detracted from the accountability of the nurse at the lowest level. Without legal status, without professional autonomy, and with a system of training which undermined professional confidence, it was unlikely that nurses in Britain would develop that professional *esprit de corps* which was necessary to foster professional accountability.

PART TWO:

Delivery of Care

Accountability in nursing models and the nursing process

3

Helen Chalmers

INTRODUCTION

Different views about the meaning of the term accountability and about its impact on nurses and nursing practice abound. The importance of the concept of accountability to the nursing profession and to the public is demonstrated in the Code of Professional Conduct for the Nurse, Midwife and Health Visitor (UKCC 1992a). The United Kingdom Central Council (UKCC) 'requires members of the professions to practise and conduct themselves within the standards and framework provided by the Code' (UKCC 1992a). Not only is it made clear that all nurses, midwives and health visitors are accountable for their practice, but all the subsequent clauses in the code hinge on the need to exercise professional accountability.

However, such a commitment by the professional body and its practitioners does not alter the fact that the idea and practice of accountability can create certain tensions among nurses. Indeed, these may be inevitable because the exercise of accountability can be very demanding, and can sometimes highlight gaps in nurses' knowledge or challenges to their usual practice. What is important is recognition of the crucial role that accountability plays in a professional group such as nurses, despite any practical or personal difficulties that may sometimes arise. It is through accountability that nurses can claim to be a profession, and it is through accountability that the profession can continue to support and develop nursing practice for the benefit of patient care.

Accountability is an inclusive term for a commitment to be responsible for any elements of nursing, such as education, management, practice and research. The purpose of this chapter is not to engage in a discussion about the multifaceted nature of accountability; rather, it is to focus on accountability in relation to practice, and in particular in relation to the way in which practice has been systematized, frequently involving the use of the nursing process, and in relation to the knowledge base underpinning practice. This is often conceptualized as a model of care. A brief resumé of these two elements of nursing practice will highlight their relevance to the notion of accountability in practice.

The nursing process

The nursing process is one way in which nurses have attempted to stylize their practice. It is a four-step problem-solving approach, not unique to nursing but nevertheless a useful aid to decision making in a variety of care settings. A large element of accountability is being able to justify what has been done and what has not been done. The nursing process and accountability share a common concern of encouraging nurses to be more conscious of the decisions they take, more aware of the care options that are available, more willing to document the decisions made and the rationales for them, and more self-questioning about the success or otherwise of action taken or omitted.

Whereas this four-step approach focuses on the process of nursing practice, models of care focus on the content, or knowledge base, necessary for safe practice. This knowledge base should not lead to routinized care but should be tailored to a person's needs. Models provide ways of thinking about nursing that highlight the need for particular kinds of knowledge and particular skills. They all share a commitment to individualized care, and at the same time they recognize that some approaches to care are more suited to certain patients than others. For example, the model of nursing developed by Peplau may not be suitable for people who are unconscious and therefore unable to communicate verbally (Peplau 1952).

Accountability, for all the tensions and difficulties it may expose, cannot be ignored by any practitioner. Indeed, it should be welcomed as it provides some recognition of the immense contribution nurses make to health care by identifying the essential relationship between nursing knowledge and skill and successful nursing interventions. Used effectively, it demonstrates that nurses are a mature professional group with the ability and willingness to take responsibility for any elements of their practice. It is more than a commitment to quality care per se: it acknowledges the need to justify actions both taken and omitted in the pursuit of quality care.

Government legislation

Clear emphasis on the role of the nurse as a skilled and knowledgeable practitioner has never been more timely. Recent government initiatives seem to demonstrate an ambiguity about the future of the nursing profession. Project 2000 was heralded as a means of preparing a more knowledgeable practitioner who would exit training with a higher education diploma as well as a nursing qualification. Project 2000 was also welcomed as a means of widening the entry gate to nursing, so that achievement in a narrow range of nationally set tests would be only one factor in the selection process. In this way the anticipated – though so far unrealized – fall in recruitment would be offset and the number of people entering the profession would be protected. Sadly, however, the numbers being recruited to nurse training are being actively reduced. This is largely because the government is strongly committed to an expanding, less qualified and more 'cost-effective' workforce.

What looks increasingly sinister for the future of high-quality nursing care is the replacement of the knowledgeable doer with the knowledgeable supervisor. Such a move, which will mean much hands-on care being provided by unqualified staff, will render accountability remote from the delivery of care. This does not bode well for professional growth and the development of nursing practice, both of which need to be vested in the delivery of care if they are to benefit patients.

In contrast, the emphasis in this chapter is on accountability which is far from remote from the essence of nursing, i.e. the delivery of nursing care. The chapter's primary focus is accountability in relation to the nursing process and models of care. For accountability to flourish in relation to direct patient care there must be professional maturity among all practitioners.

PROFESSIONAL MATURITY

This somewhat unwieldy term has been chosen to symbolize those essential attributes that nurses must bring to their practice if they are to do more than pay lip-service to the concept of accountability. Professional maturity is when a group can claim to be professional because it has a commitment to skilled practice based on knowledge; because it carries out care to a high standard; and because it is regulated by its own disciplinary body. Nurses can claim to be mature if they recognize the role they must play if they are to be called to account for their actions. Such maturity shows itself in a willingness to be self-questioning and questioned by others about the rationales for and the outcomes of acts of commission or omission, and in a willingness to celebrate those things that go well. It therefore indicates an acknowledgement of the need to be appropriately and adequately prepared in knowledge and in skill to provide high standards of care.

Knowledge and maturity

Accountability thrives in professional groups with a sound knowledge base, with a high level of skill, with a clear commitment to improving standards and with the maturity and confidence to tackle difficult decisions knowing that there will be management and professional support. Accountability flounders where there is inadequate knowledge, underdeveloped skills, little motivation, a lack of self-confidence and a fear of reprisals. The exercising of accountability is an indication of a professional group that has reached a certain maturity and values accountability as a necessary means of building on that maturity.

In order to be able to exercise accountability, nurses must be well educated and knowledgeable about nursing. Currently, the preparation to become a qualified nurse, midwife or health visitor is variable, and those already in the profession are likely to have been trained in very different ways, with different emphases in the curricula that they followed. This may not seem the most auspicious of backgrounds for a profession struggling to grasp and exploit accountability in order to benefit patient care. The issues, however, are not peculiar to nursing, nor to health-related professional groups. Changes over time are a feature of the social world. A mature profession is one that recognizes the changes taking place and one that is particularly alert to those changes that impinge upon its practice. 'Up-to-dateness' is not only about keeping abreast of developments and changes in nursing knowledge and techniques, but is also about recognizing nursing as an element of the social order, affecting and being affected by it. For example, a nurse may know about the testing of blood for the presence of human immunodeficiency virus (HIV) antibodies and may know where in a particular locality such testing is available. A limited, often medicalized, knowledge base will lead to a limited provision of advice and care which fails to take account of the impact of health-care practices on other elements of someone's life.

Professional maturity is about knowledge in a broad sense as well as about knowledge to be found in dedicated textbooks. However, it is increasingly being recognized that nurses cannot be experts in all aspects of nursing. Through its proposals for the Framework and Higher Award, the English National Board (ENB), for example, has shown itself to be committed to the development of knowledge and skills for qualified nurses that are relevant to their particular area of practice. This move should benefit nurses who are striving to be accountable by legitimizing more specialization for some practitioners.

Teamwork

The nature of nursing means that accountability exercised by nurse practitioners impinges on many in health care – the nurse, the patient, other members of the health-care team, and sometimes the family and friends of the patient. They may all be involved in the decision-making process, may all wish to consider the options available and may all have things to contribute to a process of evaluation, and may all benefit from practice developments in nursing. The UKCC has recognized the importance of collaboration and cooperation in care, and at the same time has acknowledged that difficulties can occur between members of a team. It has also, however, signalled its intention that any such conflict should 'become an influence for good' (UKCC 1989). In order for this to happen nurses and others must demonstrate a maturity of approach that ensures benefit rather than harm from any such conflict.

Professional maturity welcomes the involvement of others, rather than being threatened by it. Often the most significant contribution in the exercising of accountability comes from the patient for whose nursing care the nurse may be called to account. Recognition of the benefit to care to be gained by involving patients in the decision-making process is frequently a feature of a confident and mature health-care team which strives to individualize care and is not bound by routinized approaches.

Although the exercise of accountability is central to the role of all practitioners, there may be a place for being more specific about what accountability means for individuals. For example, nurses working in teams under the direction of a primary nurse may be accountable for different elements of practice from the primary nurse. Also, ward and unit philosophies of care might usefully include those elements of the whole for which nursing staff are accountable. This is not intended to be isolationist, but it is important that nurses, and others, recognize the limits to that for which nurses can and cannot be called to account.

Suspicion

Accountability has not been universally welcomed by nurses. To be accountable is to have responsibilities both to self and to others while having the authority to act autonomously. It can be regarded either as irksome and intrusive, or as potentiating critical thinking and professional growth. Crucially, the way in which the issue of accountability is viewed by individual practitioners, or teams of practitioners, is likely to reflect their past and present experience and their own degree of professional maturity. The greater the extent to which practitioners can see the benefits of accountability to patient care and the more confident they are in the support they get from the management of the organization in which they work, the more positive about and active in exercising accountability they will be.

Nurses have always contributed to health care in a number of ways and in a variety of settings. Changes in the structure and organization of the NHS will at times extend the role of the nurse and at other times limit it. What remains constant is the position that many nurses have in being directly involved on a day-to-day basis with patient care. In such situations nurses should welcome the opportunity to exercise accountability for the practice of nursing, and thereby demonstrate the impact of nursing on standards of care. No matter what the organizational structure, no matter what other demands are made upon them, accountability for direct patient care remains the essential key to high-quality care and to patient satisfaction with that care.

Professional maturity does not minimize the need for a recognized knowledge base from which to develop nursing care strategy. Models of nursing have recently provided a useful focus for discussion about nursing knowledge and ways in which it may differ from more medicalized understanding.

MODELS OF NURSING AND THE NURSING PROCESS

Models have gone some way towards raising nurses' awareness of the knowledge base underpinning practice. For many nurses, models of nursing have provided a welcome challenge to the medical model. For others, they have provided new ways of thinking about nursing that have, at times, been exciting and, sometimes, confusing. For some they have seemed unnecessarily complex, and for others irrelevant. At worst they have either been taken as gospel or completely dismissed; at best they have stimulated debate about the nature of people and the consequent nature of nursing.

What a model provides is a way of conceptualizing nursing that takes as its starting point the nature of people (Aggleton and Chalmers 1986). From an understanding of people, a model develops guidance on how best a person's care might be approached. Thus a model such as Orem's (1991) regards a person as someone who generally wishes to be self-caring but who, under certain circumstance, may need extensive help from nurses. Working with this model, therefore, means that nurses may be doing a considerable amount physically for a patient, and in this sense it may not seem very different from other models. What may be different, however, is the approach to care. Working with Orem's model suggests that for many people wholly compensatory nursing is unlikely to remain the best strategy of care for long. A nurse working with Orem's model should be especially alert to ways in which elements of self-care can be re-established, and to ways in which a patient can be prepared for a return to a degree of self-care. The study by Clifford (1985) points to the value of this preparatory approach in relation to ventilated patients.

The nature of nursing

Models of nursing have stimulated considerable debate about the nature of nursing. It is always valuable for ideas that broaden and deepen understanding about people and their health-care needs to be discussed and debated. When models of nursing are approached in this way they provide sets of ideas that can either challenge or support existing practice. They help to prepare the ground for the confident exercising of accountability by ensuring that nurses have thought about alternative approaches to care and can therefore explain and justify the particular way they deliver care. They do not provide a blueprint for practice, nor should they. They do, however, have an important contribution to make in nursing by focusing on the nature of people as the essential knowledge needed to underpin practice.

At the very least, nurses who are accountable cannot ignore or refute models in an unsupportable way, but must be able to justify basing care on some other set of understanding. Models of nursing or models of care form a link between being knowledgeable and being accountable.

The relationship between accountability and models of care, however, is not one that benefits from reduction to simple issues such as the value of a professed commitment to using a particular model and the existence of a set of documents seemingly demonstrating the model in use. Much more importantly, accountability provides a focus for justifying the selection of a particular model and for supporting nursing actions in relation to care. It highlights the need for decision making in nursing to be more open, more explicit and more thoughtful. A commitment to accountability makes nurses more conscious of their decision-making processes, more aware of the options to be considered, more concerned to critically evaluate care and more sensitive to the potential development of practice.

Accountability related to knowledge base and choice of model

In broad terms, in order to be able to justify working with a particular model of nursing nurses should be knowledgeable about the model and its major concepts. They cannot be exercising accountability if this is not so. They should be able to justify the model's selection for the patient or patients in their care by explaining those elements within the model that seem especially suitable. Thus, to work with Roy's model (Roy 1984), nurses must have studied the notion of adaptation and must have sufficient understanding of the biopsychosocial nature of people in order to differentiate between the four modes of adaptation described by Roy, namely the physiological, the self-concept, the role function and the interdependence modes. This demands that nurses will have explored not only the work of Roy herself, but also literature that offers additional opportunities to think through the central ideas of the model and their relevance to care. For example, the inspiration for much of Roy's model came from original research carried out by Helson (1964), who examined the influence of various types of stimuli on the human ability to adapt. In addition, there is a considerable amount of published material concerning coping strategies, a concept similar to adaptation (for example, Wilson-Barnett and Fordham 1982; Bailey and Clarke 1989).

In order to understand and discriminate between the four adaptive modes, nurses will need to have a sound understanding of physiology, psychology and social relationships and, in particular, how knowledge from these disciplines impinges on nursing care. Knowledge of the variety of ways in which adaptation or coping takes place will be crucial. For example, to care for someone with physiological needs, knowledge of control mechanisms and homoeostasis may be important in order that nurses understand how physiological balance is maintained in health and disturbed by certain stimuli. Similarly, nurses will need to be familiar with role theories and the contribution to a person's wellbeing that particular roles may make. Assessment of behaviour in the role function mode could otherwise be limited to identifying the various roles a person has rather than assessing their likely importance to the person and their care.

Accountability, in relation to working with Roy's model, also demands a sound knowledge of how people's self-concept is developed and maintained throughout life and, in particular, what threats may occur to a person's personal and physical self when they are in need of health care. In any situation in which changes to body image take place (for example pregnancy and childbirth, surgical procedures or chemotherapy), Roy's model may be especially useful as it specifically directs attention to people's concept of self and recognizes this as an important element of their nursing care.

The interdependence mode in Roy's model alerts nurses to the social nature of people. Therefore, to select the model as a guide to care demands that nurses who are accountable should be able to demonstrate an understanding of social relationships, including the ways in which they develop, change, and sometimes break down. The importance of people's social networks has been acknowledged for some time as a factor affecting health and illness, and in particular as a motivator for recovery from ill health (for example Croog and Levine 1977; Paton and Brown 1991).

At one level, accountability in relation to models of care focuses attention on a nurse's knowledge base that prepares them to implement the model. The above brief example has used Roy's model and the four adaptive modes to highlight the breadth of knowledge required. A similar picture can be elaborated for any model of care chosen to guide practice. Having selected a model, appropriate nursing skills are required for its successful implementation. Many of these skills centre on the actions taken during the stages of the nursing process.

Accountability related to the nursing process and a model of nursing

When a particular model of nursing has been selected, a systematic approach to its implementation is required. Commonly, this is the nursing process, which is essentially a problem-solving approach characterized by the four steps of assessment, planning, implementation and evaluation. The nursing process works best when seen as a circular or spiralling process, so that evaluation, for example, is integral to the process and not just the final stage. On its own, the nursing process as an approach to care is somewhat 'empty', giving nurses little more by way of guidance than that they should assess, plan, implement and evaluate. To be used in an informed manner it must be underpinned by a body of knowledge about the nature of people and the consequent nature of nursing.

What the nursing process does is focus attention on the need to be explicit about what nurses do, and it provides a framework on which to locate any elements of nursing practice. It also highlights the role and importance of documentation in nursing care as a means of recording and communicating decisions and actions taken.

If nurses claim to use the nursing process they must be able to justify its selection as an appropriate way to plan and deliver nursing care. When nursing involves identifying problems, together with ways of resolving or ameliorating them, the nursing process is probably a suitable enabling device. However, for some people in receipt of health care it may not seem the best choice. For instance, a midwife may wish to maintain an approach to care that values pregnancy, labour and childbirth as a normal event, certainly requiring involvement but not necessarily benefiting from a search for problems. Similarly, a health visitor making contact with a family with young children in order to offer health advice and screening may not be convinced about the value of an approach that focuses on a search for problems. Such difficulties may encourage the practitioner to seek an alternative process by which to approach care, or to use the nursing process in a modified form which, perhaps, seeks to identify strengths and coping skills rather than problems. In either case, the practitioner is accountable and must be able to justify the approach selected.

Assessment

When used in conjunction with a model of nursing, the nursing process, while retaining its overall four-step format, should be tailored to fit with the central tenets of the model. Assessment will always be a key feature in care when the nursing process is used. However, some models provide clear guidance about the information that should be sought at assessment, and about how it should be obtained. Some may suggest appropriate documentation as well.

An example of this is the model developed by Roper, Logan and Tierney (1990), which has found much favour among nurses in the United Kingdom. It offers an approach to care that focuses on the activities of living and acknowledges the complex influence on behaviour of factors such as sociocultural, political and economic forces, together with psychological, physical and environmental concerns. It also emphasizes the variability of human behaviour by encouraging nurses who work with the model to take account of each person's current level of activity and their own particular previous coping strategies. It recognizes the importance of nurses working within the health-care team and the complementary roles of nurses and doctors.

Working with the Roper, Logan and Tierney model, therefore, encourages the use of the nursing process in a particular way. Assessment focuses on gaining information about all 12 activities of living, including present levels of dependence and independence for each activity. Thus a nurse will seek information, for example, about an individual's ability to engage in chosen activities related to work and leisure.

Being accountable for assessment using a particular model does not mean slavishly following any given guidelines. It means that any changes which are made must be supportable, perhaps from experience or research, or perhaps from the model itself, and they must be implemented consistently.

The assessment guidelines within the Roper, Logan and Tierney model pay little attention to the influence of the various factors identified in the model and mentioned above. If, having worked with the model, a nurse or team of nurses want patient assessment to pay more attention to the influence of these factors, and can justify their importance to care planning, then it would be justifiable to incorporate them in the assessment process. Having taken this decision it would then be important to show equal commitment to each patient by consistently paying attention to factors such as economic and environmental influences when assessing their ability to be independent.

Planning and goal setting

Similarly, care planning and the setting of goals is an integral part of the nursing process used with any model of nursing. There is currently considerable pressure to make all goals patient-centred. Although this is generally to be welcomed as a means of ensuring that care planning goes beyond identifying what nurses should do, and rightly focuses attention on patient outcomes, an accountable nurse working with Peplau's model (Peplau 1952), for example, might justify a somewhat different approach. Peplau's model emphasizes the human ability to develop throughout life, and sees all experience as an opportunity, through interpersonal relationships, for people to develop further or in different ways. Thus, Peplau sees episodes in someone's life involving contact with a nurse as providing opportunities for development both for the person and for the nurse. Using this model it would be appropriate to have nurse-centred goals in addition to those that identify patient outcomes.

Nurses working with most models of nursing will find that the setting of short- and long-term goals is advocated. Some models may even suggest intermediate goals as well. For many patients this is appropriate. Nevertheless, there may be occasions when a patient's particular circumstances indicate that care might best be managed by using an interactionist model and short-term goals only. One feature of models that draw on interactionist theory, such as that developed by Riehl-Sisca (1989), is that they define all action as meaningful to the person undertaking it. There may be times when such an approach is valuable for a patient whose behaviour is proving challenging to the care team. Traditional, and often medicalized, models tend to focus on trying to eliminate or subdue behaviour when what is needed is a commitment and an opportunity to try and understand the meaning of the behaviour from the patient's point of view.

With this commitment in mind, nurses working with an interactionist model may find themselves unable to set achievable goals other than short-term ones. Trying to define the meaning of someone's behaviour when it seems to be at odds with social norms is both difficult and time-consuming. It is only as ater understanding emerges over time that more goals can be set. The rse–patient relationship may always be developing, making it unlikely that ore than short-term goals can be identified, especially if there is to be patient volvement with, and agreement to, goals set whenever possible.

Intervention

The third stage of the nursing process relies on the information obtained during assessment and on the careful planning for care that goes along with it. Intervention is the central part of nursing. It is that part of the process where nurses use their skills in order to aid the patient in the achievement of goals. As with any skilled work, much of nursing looks deceptively simple to an outside observer who knows little about the knowledge required or the essential skills. Indeed, much of nursing may seem uncomplicated to a nurse when they have developed into an expert practitioner. It is crucial that nurses do not underestimate their own knowledge and skills. If they do they are likely to increase the numbers of unqualified staff who cannot provide the same quality of care.

Accountability can help us to value nursing interventions because it goes beyond acknowledging that certain things have been done in accordance with a plan of care. It focuses attention on why something was done, why it was done in a particular way, why some additional intervention took place at the same time and on the continuing role of assessment during intervention.

Those who support an increasingly unqualified workforce may claim that, as long as assessment and care planning are carried out by a qualified nurse, the quality of care will not suffer. Such a notion is only compatible with a linear view of the nursing process, which sees assessment as a one-off or, at best, periodic process.

During all nursing interventions, and every contact with patients, qualified nurses are in a position to continually update and add to their understanding of patients and their needs. In order to demonstrate this, nurses must be diligent about documenting changes to care in the light of the developing nature of their assessment. Such a commitment is essential if nurses are to demonstrate accountability for the dynamic nature of nursing practice.

All models require that nurses have a range of skills to choose from in the intervention stage of the nursing process. In order to be accountable for care, using any model, nurses must be satisfied that they have gained the requisite skills to an appropriate level.

In order to be registered practitioners, nurses must have reached a required level of skill that will equip them to work with any model to a certain level. However, some models may emphasize the value of particular skills to a higher level in the provision of high-quality care. Accountability, in this circumstance, may encourage nurses to update their skills or to develop them further. For example, in Riehl's model of nursing (Riehl-Sisca 1989) there is a special need for interactional skills. Based on symbolic interactionism, Riehl's model relies not only on more traditional strategies but also on nurses having skills to intervene in ways that may not feature in initial training. A nurse working with Riehl's model might encourage a patient to engage in role-taking or in role-play, perhaps in order to help them to begin to come to terms with a necessary change in lifestyle. This might, for instance, help someone who has had a coronary thrombosis to think through the benefits and difficulties of taking more exercise and changing their eating habits. Such strategies demand that nurses have the skills to encourage the patient to think about a change in lifestyle, or to try out new behaviours in a safe setting. Of equal importance is the need for skills that will enable nurses to debrief the patient sensitively and effectively after implementing a plan of care.

Within Orem's model (Orem 1991) there is a clear commitment to an educative role for the nurse. Although teaching skills are needed when working with any model, an accountable practitioner working with this model is likely to feel the need for more developed teaching skills, so that the crucial role envisaged by Orem can be effective. A recognition of this need may lead the practitioner to investigate suitable educational courses and to make a case to management for support to attend such a course. Ideally, a nurse should be able to gain the necessary skills for working with a particular model with the support of management. Accountable practice demands the acquisition of appropriate skills and, while it is the individual practitioner's responsibility to ensure that they have the skills, they have a corresponding right to practical support from management, such as study time and help with tuition fees.

Decision making about nursing intervention must be based on knowledge, tempered by the particular circumstances that prevail. It may mean, for example, that knowledge in one sphere may conflict with other available information, making the choice of action uncertain. Knowledge of the hazards of smoking may at times be at odds with the knowledge of someone's deliberate choice and their right to continue smoking.

There are many occasions when health education advice may conflict with a chosen lifestyle, and while this does not obviate the responsibility to give appropriate advice, it does point to the need for a sensitive approach that acknowledges its own limitations. In such a circumstance, the nature of accountability is reasonably clear. Offering a person up-to-date information about the dangers of smoking is justifiable on the basis of current pathophysiological knowledge. Intervention, however, should not extend to removing cigarettes from an individual who wishes to continue to smoke. A nurse may therefore be called to account for the provision of health education advice but should not be called to account for failing to make an individual stop smoking.

The nursing process used with a model of care offers an approach to nursing care that make possible this integrative use of different arenas of knowledge (such as pathophysiology and personal choice). Once a commitment is made to patient involvement with those aspects of care to which they wish and are able to contribute, nurses have access to the special arena of knowledge that centres on patients' rights and individual choice. It is crucial that nurses can demonstrate that they have accessed this knowledge if they are to be accountable for individualized care.

Evaluation

For convenience, the evaluation stage of the nursing process is considered last, although when practitioners are exercising accountability formative evaluation will be going on throughout the delivery of care. This is essential in order for the nursing process to assist nurses in their efforts to remain sensitive to changes in what patients need during a span of care. Thoughtful, accountable practice will often be exemplified by alterations and adjustments to planned care made in the light of such evaluation.

For example, a patient who has difficulty in walking following a prolonged period in bed, may negotiate goals that expect only limited progress in the first few days. Very often, people lack confidence after a period of dependency and it is usually counterproductive to set goals that they feel are unmanageable. People's confidence may be boosted more effectively if they discover that their progress has exceeded their own expectations. In such a circumstance the nurse must be able to explain the setting of limited goals, and will require opportunities to evaluate progress frequently so that new goals can reflect the patient's increased confidence and mobility. The interface between formative evaluation, reassessment and sensitive, appropriate goal setting is crucial, and demands the knowledge, skills and commitment of qualified, accountable practitioners.

Formative evaluation is likely to draw on information from a variety of sources, in particular the opinions, feelings and behaviour of the patient. For care to remain dynamic and relevant, nurses must be diligent in their efforts to make sense of all the information available about a patient's nursing care. Sometimes a remark from a relative, a concern expressed by a care assistant or an observation that does not quite fit the expected pattern will signal the need for prompt evaluation and reassessment of care.

The ideas underpinning particular models of care will provide a focus and direction for evaluation by emphasizing certain aspects of the nature of people. Orem's model of nursing (Orem 1991) values the self-care abilities of people. A thoughtful commitment to this model might encourage nurses to develop a format for evaluation that gives patients the opportunity to carry out significant parts of the evaluative process themselves. This might involve designing a semistructured evaluation questionnaire for patients to fill in periodically, or might involve some patients writing a brief daily report on their perception of their progress. Other patients might be able to discuss how they feel about the care they are receiving and describe any movement toward goal attainment during nursing staff handover, or to the nurse accountable for their care.

Orem (1991) also identifies a key role for people who are significant to the patient (this will sometimes be the patient's family) when the patient is unable to be self-caring. Accountable practice, in this instance, may be demonstrated by the nurse approaching such significant people in order to gain their help in the evaluative process. Some of the strategies identified above may still be suitable with some modifications. For example, a partner or spouse may be willing to write a brief daily report during a visit to the patient, or in time for a community nurse's call.

Summative evaluation has a somewhat broader emphasis and holds the key to the development of practice through experience and reflection. Accountability is not just about being able to adequately support current practices; it is also about being committed to developing practice so that care strategies do not stagnate but remain sensitive to changes in knowledge, whether discovered through the literature or learned through practice itself.

A genuine commitment to reflect on a particular patient's care, or on experience gained by working with a model of nursing over a period of time, is crucial. Very often, this careful thinking through of what was done and the outcomes of action taken is best carried out in teams. In order to be effective it requires documentation of a high quality, where an accurate account of what took place is recorded, so that it can be examined. Things do not always go according to plan in health care and, while this is rarely desirable, it does provide an opportunity for a careful assessment and evaluation of what went right and what went wrong. It is necessary to question what took place and to develop practice by reflecting on which strategies were successful and on how care could be improved.

Accountability, therefore, is not about things always going right, although it is about making decisions that can be supported. It is about being able to justify what was done and, when things go wrong, being able to take account of what happened to ensure that lessons are learned and that practice develops.

Where a working climate and environment have developed in which careful summative evaluation of care is the norm, nursing records may improve. Nurses who select a patient as a subject for a written care study often indicate that their care plans benefit in terms of information, recorded because they know that only with reliable information can they engage in a careful analysis and evaluation of care. Knowing that a summative evaluation will take place, and that documentation will be an important source of information, may similarly improve the recording of nursing care delivered and its rationale. Better written sources of patient information hold the potential to improve care by ensuring that those involved in care provision are more adequately informed.

In some instances accountability, particularly when linked to summative evaluation, can strengthen the demand for clearly focused nursing research. Evaluation that raises repeated doubts about the appropriateness of action taken may lead to a more formal examination of practice.

ENVIRONMENT OF SUPPORT

In order for any professional group to accept the principle of accountability, there must be both a secure and appropriate knowledge base and sufficient maturity to recognize the potential advantage of exercising accountability, as well as the difficulties that may occur.

Managers, whether they are nurses or not, while recognizing that nurses are bound to exercise accountability if they are to conform to their code of professional conduct, should help them to see accountability as something positive and useful, and not as an unwelcome adjunct to practice. They can do this in a number of ways, but in particular by taking note of information generated by the exercise of accountability and by supporting nurses' efforts to use this information to improve practice. Sometimes such support may be in terms of different resources, or agreement to new working practices. Managers must be prepared to listen to nurses when they express concerns about issues of quality that have the sound backing of meaningful data gathered during practice. Nurses must be open about their concerns and conscientious in ensuring that data gathered are valid and reliable. They must try to go beyond highlighting anxieties by offering realistic proposals for change.

Change

Accountability thus provides the opportunity to support existing practice and also provides a vehicle for change. It can support or challenge knowledge. It can highlight the usefulness of certain skills or demonstrate the need to develop new ones. It can and should stimulate nurses to develop practice. Unfortunately, it can also alienate nurses and managers by seeming over-complex and demanding. This latter situation is increasingly common where nurses feel undervalued by managers and lack management support, or where managers have been unconvinced of the importance of accountability because nurses have failed to demonstrate its role in the provision of high-quality care.

The exercising of accountability thrives in an atmosphere of support, challenge, encouragement, mutual respect and trust. To be accountable frequently demands that difficult questions are asked, and there must be a climate for working that facilitates this. There must be adequate systems to support any rational and legitimate action that is taken as a result of nurses' commitment to being accountable.

Nursing needs to take place in an organization where managers, as well as nurses, recognize the enormous variability of human behaviour, and where this recognition fosters creative, flexible and non-routinized systems of care. For nurses to act autonomously they must be active creators and negotiators of care initiatives. They cannot be passive, nor can they be isolated from the mainstream of practice, where debate about care strategies and the outcomes of nursing interventions go hand in hand with accountability.

Managers can often demonstrate understanding of the complex nature of accountability by recognizing the need for nurses to have regular time set aside to reflect upon summative evaluations of patient care, in order to make recommendations for ways in which standards could be improved. Nurses must demonstrate their commitment to accountability and to the organization in which they work, by making sure that such time is well spent and that realistic and useful recommendations are made.

Crucially, accountability should provide nurses themselves, and the public, with confidence in the quality of nursing care. The potential for benefit to patient care due to the thoughtful exercise of accountability within a climate of support is immense.

CONCLUSION

Acceptance of the need for and the benefits of accountability provides an exciting stimulus for nurses to keep up to date. Motivation by such measures is infinitely preferable to mandatory requirements for practitioners to update themselves, and in this way nurses benefit from learning that is meaningful, self-generated and self-valuing.

During a period of major upheaval in the management of the NHS, the future direction and influence of nursing is in the balance. This provides an opportunity for nurses to reflect upon what has been and what now might be. For many nurses, the direct involvement with day-to-day care is the essence of nursing. It has never been more important to convince others of the vital role that suitably qualified nurses play in the provision of high-quality care. Used effectively, accountability is an ideal means of demonstrating the unique contribution made by nurses.

In order to achieve such recognition nurses themselves must be convinced of their own value to patient care and must be able to clearly identify the boundaries of nursing. They must be prepared and able to justify what they do and what they do not do in ways that others can understand and appreciate. Curtin, writing more than 10 years ago (Curtin 1982), saw the major battle for the acceptance of accountability to be among nurses themselves. If this battle has now been won, then a significant hurdle has been crossed in the struggle to get nurses themselves to value nursing and to value their role as accountable practitioners.

Standards of care, quality assurance and accountability

4

Lesley Duff

INTRODUCTION

It is apparent from the subject matter of this volume that the concept of account-ability is multifaceted and complex. This complexity is further compounded when accountability is considered in relation to an evolving professionalism in nursing and the changes that this entails for nurses in their responsibilities, authority and autonomy. This chapter will consider fully where the responsibil-ity for accountability lies by comparing and contrasting the processes of disclo-sure and recounting. In short, recounting is initiated by others, whereas disclosure is initiated by the individual and in this way more accurately encap-sulates the notion of accountability.

In the course of this chapter I aim to suggest how the techniques of quality assurance can be used to implement accountability in the care settings in which most nurses work, to explain why these techniques can be so used and to consider some of the dilemmas that face nurses who embrace accountability and try to make it work.

For the purpose of trying to put into operation the concept of accountability I have chosen to use the definition given by Pembrey (1992) in the introduction to her seminar on the relationship between the professional's role and their responsibility given at the National Institute of Nursing, Oxford. This definition is a distillation of a definition developed by Lewis and Batey (1982a,b) in their review of the subject, in which accountability is defined as a) to be answerable, and b) the fulfilment of a formal obligation to disclose to referent others matters relating to that for which one has authority. The information contained within these definitions gives us a starting point for exercising accountability in practice. In order to be answerable, we need something to be answerable for and someone to whom we are answerable.

DISCLOSURE

Disclosure is the process of making visible information which is relevant to the situation for which we have responsibility or authority. It includes everything, from the purpose of activities carried out through to the expenditures involved. The content of the disclosure reveals and explains how responsibilities have been discharged, and its purpose is to enable decisions and evaluations to be made. A disclosure involves discretion on the part of the person making the disclosure about its timing and its scope or depth. Initiation of the disclosure is the responsibility of the accountable person, and not those to whom the disclosure is being made.

This control of the procedure of disclosure helps us to interpret what accountability is in a practical sense, as distinct from simple recounting of what has been done. Freed (1975) describes recounting as what the nursing service does retrospectively and defensively in order to explain nurses' acts. Recounting is initiated by others; it carries the implication of error, and it occurs when people are called to task and asked to recreate and justify their actions, plans and goals. When recounting occurs, norms or organizational guidelines are perceived to have been violated. Accounting, by contrast, implies that the person making the disclosure has both authority and autonomy in the areas of responsibility. To be accountable denotes an acceptance of the obligation to disclose and of the possible consequences of disclosure.

Considering accountability and disclosure in this detail gives rise to a new set of questions:

- Who are the referent others?
- What are we answerable for, i.e. for what do we have authority?
- How can we make a formal disclosure about what we do?

Referent others

The referent others for nurses can be one of a number of groups of people:

- the patients or clients;
- other colleagues within the profession;
- other colleagues outside the profession of nursing;
- the organization within which the nurse works.

In other words, anyone with a vested interest in the information to be disclosed because of their need to make decisions or to set policy on the basis of that information.

The question of who the referent others are is the crux of how accountability is implemented in nursing. Internal and external mechanisms exist to allow access to these referent others and for disclosure to take place.

Traditionally, the regulation of nurses has been carried out by an external mechanism, first the General Nursing Council (GNC) and then the United Kingdom Central Council for Nursing, Midwifery and Health Visiting (UKCC). These bodies have very much acted as custodians of the public interest by maintaining and controlling a register, with the power to remove people from that register, together with their right to practise. Latterly the UKCC has moved more towards the view that the external regulatory agent should also help to foster internal regulation by practitioners. This is demonstrated in the latest edition of the code of conduct, to which all nurses on the register must adhere (UKCC 1992a). In this document the major line of accountability for nurses – that is, the dominant group of referent others – is emphasized as being to the patients. It does not deny that lines of accountability exist between nurses and their colleagues and the organizations they work for but, as Pyne (1992) states, 'the lines in the other directions are dotted lines rather than solid lines, or at least of fainter hue'. This represents the transition taking place in nursing whereby the UKCC is encouraging nurses to see themselves as accountable to the people they care for, while retaining its role as a referent other for the purposes of disclosure. The use of terms such as 'lines of accountability' demonstrate how accountability is seen as being achieved through a hierarchy, which begins with the patient and travels through colleagues and the employing organization to the UKCC itself.

For what do we have authority?

The answer to this question hinges on the clarification of the complexity of the issues involved in understanding accountability, which are determined by the related concepts of responsibility and autonomy as well as by the notion of accountability itself.

Responsibility

Responsibility is defined by Lewis and Batey (1982a) as a charge for which one is responsible, and can derive from external or internal sources. Nurses have traditionally accepted charges from external sources, whether they were carrying out the instructions of a doctor or the ward sister, and the discharge of these responsibilities has traditionally been unquestioning. Nursing has also assumed charges that are not perceived by those outside nursing as legitimate responsibilities.

There is currently a development taking place whereby nursing is reviewing the services it offers to patients and looking at ways of defining the goals of those services, specifying the procedures it will use to achieve those goals, and conducting evaluation studies to determine outcomes. Such clarity of position is essential if nursing is to continue to develop and to gain understanding of the relationship between personal autonomy and accountability.

Authority

Authority is not inherent in responsibility but derives from at least three sources.

Authority of expert knowledge

This exists when society grants the rightful power to assume certain responsibilities through a licence or a place on a register. An example of this is the register held by the UKCC of practitioners eligible to practise. Registration follows either examinations or acceptance following various access routes stipulated by the UKCC for nurses qualifying overseas, and is accompanied by the individual's receipt of a document entitled *The Scope of Professional Practice*. This outlines the responsibilities that a registered nurse can be expected to fulfil as well as the knowledge and skills needed to carry them out.

The present state of flux in nursing is illustrated by the recent changes in this UKCC document (UKCC 1992b). Previously it was the case that nursing was seen as a specific set of activities and responsibilities, with anything extra being referred to as the 'extended role of the nurse'. The power to carry out these activities was granted by the employing body on the basis of a certificate of competence. Now these 'extended role' activities are subsumed in the general expected responsibilities of the nurse. The decision about whether a nurse has the necessary skills and knowledge to carry out the responsibilities as outlined in *The Scope of Professional Practice* lies with the nurse.

An example of one such task is the giving of intravenous drugs. It used to be the case that anyone who passed a certificated test for their administration could give these drugs, that is, they could assume the charge or responsibility to give them. The certificate did not indicate their competence to do so but rather the permission of the employing body, evidenced by the fact that the certificates were not transferable between employing bodies. The authority of nurses to give the drugs was unclear, as the knowledge base from which they discharged the responsibility of giving them was slight. The authority was therefore not that of the nurse on the basis of their expert knowledge. How then could a nurse be called to account for this task, beyond reporting to a supervisor?

The authority of knowledge goes beyond the minimum standards expressed by statute or regulation. Peplau (1971) states that 'the more explanatory knowledge a nurse has and can use the more likely she is to have fewer problems in authority connected with practice responsibilities which she takes'. The same holds for nursing as a collective body. Such explanatory knowledge need not be unique to nursing, but as nursing formulates and tests theories relevant to its practice it will be in a stronger position to assert its authority derived from expert knowledge.

Kitson (1993) supports this assertion when considering the move from strict guidelines and hierarchies in nursing practice. She believes that unless practices can be defended on clinical effectiveness or properly conducted research studies, it is questionable whether the nurse is acting responsibly in continuing to carry them out.

Situational authority

A second source of authority is that of the situation. In an emergency, for example, the rightful power to fulfil what needs to be done is accorded to those present, even though in non-emergency conditions such power would not normally exist.

Positional authority

The third source of authority described by Lewis and Batey (1982a) is the authority of position. This is the rightful power to act which is tied to a formal position, and specifically to an individual. Stevens (1976) calls this administrative authority. Some of the conflicts that occur regarding authority appear in situations where nurses are given responsibility for something but no authority to actually carry it out. In other words, there is no authority linked to the position in which the nurse is employed, and related to this is the concept of autonomy.

Autonomy and authority

The term autonomy is used variably to mean self-determination or self-direction, to be able to design a total plan of care and to interact on an independent level with other professionals, and not to have one's behaviour controlled by an external agent.

Hall (1968) distinguishes two characteristics of autonomy, the attitudinal and the structural. Structural autonomy exists when professional people are expected to use their judgement to determine the provision of client services in the context of their work. Attitudinal autonomy exists for people who believe themselves to be free to exercise judgement in decision making. Engel (1970) further clarified this by defining work-related autonomy as the freedom of the professional to practise in accordance with their professional training. A synthesis of these meanings and conditions gives a definition of autonomy which is the freedom to make discretionary and binding decisions consistent with one's scope of practice and the freedom to act on these decisions (Lewis and Batey 1982a).

Discretionary decisions are those based on up-to-date and extensive knowledge about the subject and judgements involving comprehensive investigations into the means by which to reach goals. Once a decision has been made it is binding, in so much as it is owned by the professional, and as such cannot be altered by anyone else except through discussion. Autonomy and authority are, thereby, linked when the scope of practice is defined. Autonomy is not just about decision-making but also about the authority to act on any decision made. Authority is defined as the rightful power to fulfil a responsibility, and autonomy is the freedom to exercise that power. This freedom derives from two sources: from organizational structure and from the individual professional. This 'willingness' to be autonomous, however, can mean that nurses are often their own worst enemies (Thompson 1967; Pembrey 1992).

Organizations can influence individuals' willingness to exercise autonomy and make discretionary decisions by their sanctioning structure. The structure of the organization affects autonomy by the power of veto. As long as another unit of the organization can legitimately exercise the power of veto over decisions autonomy cannot exist. This has implications when we come to look at how disclosures are made.

The principal consequence of autonomy is accountability: whoever has autonomy must be answerable for its inherent freedom. Decisions and actions in the context of autonomy are the professional's own and cannot be shifted to another when the outcomes are less than favourable.

How can we make a formal disclosure?

We can see from the discussion so far that how we make a formal disclosure is dependent on whether we are operating within the mechanisms of external or internal regulation, and therefore to which group of referent others we make the disclosure. In external regulation the 'how' of disclosure is defined by a system in which there is a set of guidelines or protocols to which the nurse must adhere. How well this adherence is achieved is ascertained by exercising a system of hierarchical accountability, for example the supervision of a nurse carrying out the activity needed to discharge a responsibility, by someone with more authority. The role of the night sister is a good illustration of this. The night sister in traditional settings provides the expertise necessary to supervise the nurses working at night, sometimes in situations in which a more senior nurse might be employed in the daytime. Other external regulating mechanisms make use of the employer–employee relationship, or the maintenance of a licensing system or register.

There is only a limited sense in which a nurse can, in any way, be said to be accountable for the discharge of responsibilities based on a plan of action and protocols decided by someone else. The nurse lacks the necessary authority and autonomy. As described in the introduction, accounting contrasts markedly with recounting. The fulfilment of accountability involves a systematic and periodic disclosure about that for which a person is answerable, which is initiated and controlled by the person making the disclosure.

Internal regulation takes place through such mechanisms as peer review, the development of personal and professional accountability and by professional supervision. The role of the consultant with the junior doctor demonstrates how different this form of supervision is from that of the old-fashioned night sister. The consultant supervises the activities of junior staff by acting as a kind of mentor. Junior doctors are accountable for their care of a patient and determine their own plans of care. However, the consultant has the power, by virtue of authority, to veto any decisions made. The supervision appears to be more in the form of advice and access to expertise than the prescription of activities to be monitored by senior staff. In such a situation the disclosure takes the form of a discussion of the ways in which the junior doctor intends to act, or of the way in which they have acted, with the tacit agreement that the consultant has the right of veto as described above. The actual carrying out of supervision in this way can be more or less formal, depending on the style of the doctors taking part. Rarely, however, will a junior doctor be asked to recount their exercise of a procedure in a way that implies they had no involvement in determining that the procedure should be used.

In this scenario the junior doctor does not have full autonomy, but autonomy within the defined parameters of their expertise. They are accountable for the decisions regarding the care given, but the consultant is also partly accountable through the exercise of their supervisory function.

Primary nursing is an example of how a similar system can exist in nursing, and this is discussed in more detail in Chapter 5. In primary nursing, nurses determine the plan of care for their patients. The senior nurse on the ward or unit is available for advice, and has the power of veto over any plans drawn up. The veto should be exercised through discussion and the use of scientific evidence if any of the plans are to be challenged. The primary nurse, in turn, supervises the execution of the care plans by associate nurses. In this scenario the primary nurse is accountable for the care of the patient and the associate nurse is accountable to the primary nurse for their part in the discharge of the responsibilities connected with that care. Who, then, is the referent other for the primary nurse? The patient is said to be the prime referent other but there are rarely mechanisms in place for this to be a reality. More usually the nurse would make disclosure to peers, perhaps in the course of a ward meeting or case conference, or through professional review mechanisms such as appraisal or individual performance review. In nursing, the hierarchical accountability system also remains in place in most establishments, but it could be that through the gradual process of change the move towards internal regulation will become complete.

Each of these approaches has implications for how we understand and carry out accountability in practice. By following a purely external regulatory model we are accountable only to the person above us in the hierarchy. We may adhere to the protocols set out for the discharge of a responsibility, but as the protocols have been determined by someone else, with more authority than we have, and because we will have to demonstrate that we have fulfilled the requirements or the protocols, we can in no way be said to be accountable for what we do. The truth of the matter is, as highlighted by Lewis and Batey's definition (1982a,b), that accountability is related more to demonstrable levels of competency, skills and knowledge, and having the confidence that comes from experience and up-to-date knowledge to decide what has to be done and how to do it, than to the successful completion of a task. Without being instrumental in the design of a task the nurse is only a contributory factor in discharging the responsibility of someone who does have the necessary authority, skills and knowledge. The nurse must then abide within the hierarchical system set up to protect the interests of the person with ultimate accountability. Where, then, does that leave nurses in their pursuit of professional recognition and the assumptions of accountability that go with it?

PUTTING ACCOUNTABILITY INTO OPERATION

The transition from external to internal mechanisms of regulation is not easy. Consider the consequences of moving to decision-making outside the strict guidelines afforded by rigid protocols and hierarchical structures. Each point in the delivery of a service involves an overwhelming number of choices. How much is even known about the effectiveness of many of the nursing interventions to which these choices relate? Again, this emphasizes the need for properly conducted research in order to evaluate clinical practice for its effectiveness, but it also suggests a need for a structured approach to capturing nursing knowledge which allows it to be critically evaluated and disseminated. There is a similar problem in medicine (Smith 1991), perhaps compounded by a reluctance on the part of some doctors to acknowledge that there are any uncertainties in medical practice (N. Black 1992) and to share evaluative information.

Nursing can perhaps learn from medicine, where professionalism is the cherished norm and internal regulation assumed and defended at all costs as a defence against potential legal action and loss of power.

The move toward personal accountability is complemented by a need for the development of clearer research-based protocols, or standards outlining best practice. This should not be perceived as a move back to a system of external regulation, but instead as a way in which the individual nurse, in consultation with peers, can describe in a constructive way what best practice is in a particular area. Nurses can then decide whether they have sufficient skill and expertise to take the lead in planning, coordinating and delivering nursing care to the patient. This is a very important point in the development of nurses as autonomous practitioners. There is a certain suspicion on the part of colleagues and managers that nurses do not have the knowledge base or sufficiently researched practices to assume responsibility outside the safety guards of strict guidelines or protocols. The need for rigorously researched practices with defined outcomes cannot, in this context, be stressed enough. The prerequisites for accountability, responsibility, authority and, in consequence autonomy, depend on it.

If something untoward happens, the existence of such protocols or standards also demonstrates that professional accountability has been exercised through a consideration of the activities and roles involved in the discharge of a particular responsibility. Public accountability is made possible through the clear presentation of responsibilities undertaken, the level of competence expected and the expected outcomes. Significantly, it is this feature of defining care in the form of a standard which sometimes makes nurses nervous, the concern being that they may put themselves at greater risk legally by making explicit certain outcomes of care they wish to achieve, or by specifying how exactly they intend to act.

How to delineate spheres of responsibility and how to gain autonomy: techniques of quality assurance

The development and use of protocols and standards by the professionals who intend to use them as the delineation of best practice is very much akin to the developments within quality assurance (QA) in nursing. Here there has been a gradual shift towards nurses assuming responsibility for changing their practice in the light of self and peer audit. Generated by a similar shift in thinking to that driving the move towards professionalism and the pragmatic dictates of activating change, this approach to QA is best represented in the United Kingdom by the system developed by the Royal College of Nursing (RCN), known as the dynamic standard-setting system (RCN 1990).

The standards used for the purposes of QA can be written by experts outside the area in which they will be used, and applied by an external assessor, or they may be set by the nurses themselves to define their goals and how they intend to achieve them. The standards represent overall yardsticks against which practice can be evaluated. Myriad definitions are used for standards and the related concept of criteria. The RCN (1990) uses the term to mean 'a professionally agreed level of performance for a particular population, which is achievable, observable, desirable, and measurable'. Criteria provide the more detailed practical information on how a particular standard is to be achieved, and can be described (RCN 1990) as the 'items or variables selected as indicators of the quality of care'.

There is considerable debate about who should formulate and apply the standards and criteria. Two main schools of thought have emerged in the last 20 years which are reflective of the changes in nursing and its status as an autonomous internally regulated profession. The first can be considered to be the traditional view, which sees QA as a method of controlling the quality of the product produced by concentrating on the identification and removal of apparently poor performers through the application of externally derived standards. The alternative view is that of applying QA techniques to identify opportunities for improvement, which are then activated by staff development and the introduction of change.

Nursing currently uses both approaches to QA. Predetermined tools representative of the traditional approach were developed throughout the 1960s, 1970s and early 1980s, and include those such as Monitor (Goldstone *et al.* 1983), Qualpacs (Wandelt and Ager 1974), and the Phaneuf Nursing Audit (Phaneuf 1976). Throughout this same period national nurses' associations, particularly in North America and Australia, were active in producing national standards and guidelines for practice. However, experiences of implementing traditional quality assurance systems have been varied, and recent research has highlighted the importance of concepts such as employee participation, involvement and control throughout the implementation period (Harvey 1991). A lack of involvement is more often associated with negative feelings towards assessment, such as feelings of anxiety, defensiveness and threat akin to those engendered by the process of recounting, and indeed recounting may be employed in some traditional methods of QA. Such discomfort on the part of practitioners can give rise to the attitude that QA, and the whole mechanism of accountability, only exists to exert control over the people working within an organization, rather than a perception that it can be a valuable method of enhancing the quality of service. Once such an attitude is established it can be very difficult to keep sight of the purpose of having such systems, namely the enhancement of the quality of care given to patients, the ultimate referent others.

From the 1980s onwards there has been an increasing interest in involving nurses, or practitioners of other disciplines, as the key to achieving lasting and meaningful change. The unit-based approach of Shroeder and Maibusch (1984) and the dynamic standard-setting system are examples of this. In these methods ownership and control is devolved to the level of service delivery, and practitioners themselves are responsible for defining the standards and criteria against which their practice is to be compared. This demonstrates the philosophy on which these approaches are based – that is, that all those involved in the care of the patient are an essential and valued part of the total experience. This philosophy means that everyone involved in giving care is expected to contribute to decisions regarding that care, both in setting standards and in evaluating care by means of those standards. By using such an approach to QA it is felt that nurses are empowered to accept full responsibility for quality and to function more proactively in its pursuit.

Comparing this philosophy with the prerequisites of accountability outlined at the beginning of the chapter, it can be clearly seen that standard setting can be a useful way of fulfilling the determinants of each.

Responsibility

When a group of nurses come together to look at an area of care they will first decide whether the subject they want to look at is something within their sphere of responsibility and something they can do something about if there are indications for change. If the subject is within their sphere of responsibility as defined by the UKCC code of conduct (UKCC 1992a) they will then consider whether it is something which concerns only their professional group, or whether any decisions made have implications for colleagues. If the subject only concerns nurses they can go ahead with the standard setting; if not, they need to set the standards along with other colleagues involved in that area of care. Nutrition is a good example of this. If the concern is that patients are not receiving a hot meal, the nurses may need to work on the standard with representatives of the portering service. If the standard concerns the positioning of patients at mealtimes the nurses may take advice from a physiotherapist but then write the standard themselves.

Standards written using a practitioner-based approach make explicit the composite nature of the care to be given, particularly if a structured approach such as the dynamic standard-setting system is used. Standards in this format comprise a statement which outlines the broad objective or goal of implementation, followed by three criteria sets which define what is needed for the achievement of the standard: structure and process criteria, and what the outcome of implementing the standard should be. This serves the dual purpose of allowing the standard to be both implemented and audited, because the criteria indicate by their presence or absence whether or not the standard has been reached. This in turn enables improvements to be made to care, as it is clear where shortfalls are occurring on one criterion or another.

The nurses may decide to adopt a standard written by someone else, but the same consideration of the procedures should be made by those who will implement the standard. The purpose of this is twofold. First, it makes clear whether the procedures needed to achieve a particular standard can be implemented within the constraints of a particular situation, and secondly it allows the nurses to decide whether they have the necessary skills and knowledge to discharge the responsibilities the standard represents. If nurses write their own standards they will be written to accommodate the skills and knowledge of the group writing them.

Authority

As authority relates to the knowledge base and the power to exercise it that is held by the professional, the setting of standards by the group who intend to use them is a valuable way of taking back power from those who set standards externally. The very fact that nurses are given the freedom to set their own standards is an important first step to claiming authority, but it is not the whole story.

Also important is the fact that nurses can then take charge of the whole process of disclosure by the audit of those standards, and can make changes as a result of this process.

Audit is the term used to describe the evaluation of practice against the standards set, whether by the professionals themselves or externally (RCN 1993a). In the dynamic standard-setting system and other methods that give control of the audit activity back to nurses, the standard acts as the blueprint for the audit, with the criteria becoming the quality indicators. The nurses carry out the audit or make the decision to employ the services of an external auditor. They evaluate the results and draw up action plans to remedy any shortfall identified.

In some institutions an organizational structure will have been set up to review these QA and audit activities. Often, there will be an audit committee to which the nurses may make presentations of their work or send reports. In this way the nurses can control the disclosure of information about their activities, a fact they may exploit by using the disclosure situation to negotiate, for example for funding or changes to a staffing rota. Without a well defined structure for disclosing the results of audit this can be more difficult, but it is still possible for the nurses to take charge of the disclosure process by enlisting the support of their managers before they begin.

By giving nurses the responsibility to carry out audit and change against self-determined standards in this way, there is inherent acknowledgement by their peers and management that they have the legitimate authority as a group to accept such responsibility. It is, therefore, a first step to replacing organizational accountability – an external mechanism of regulation – with an internal mechanism, peer review. This accords well with the move towards developing nurses as more autonomous and therefore accountable practitioners, and fulfils in part the curious anomaly that a person cannot actually become accountable for something until or unless they have been publicly acknowledged as being capable of taking on that accountability. This anomaly arises from Lewis and Batey's (1982a,b) definition, which requires three other factors to be in place if accountability is to be achieved: i) responsibility, i.e. the charge for which a person is responsible; ii) authority, i.e. having the rightful expertise and power to fulfil that charge; and iii) autonomy, i.e. having the freedom to decide what to do and to do it.

As described above, however, setting and auditing your own standards is not the whole story. Standard setting allows the demarcation of legitimate responsibilities. How can this be successfully carried out when a group may be willing to take part in the exercise but experience great resistance from colleagues in other professions? The slow acceptance of clinical audit illustrates this point and demonstrates the difficulty that nurses have in being accepted by their colleagues as truly accountable for what they do.

Clinical audit is a method by which all professionals involved in an area of care come together to define their objectives for that care and to set joint standards for the achievement of those objectives. The care given is then evaluated, or audited, against these standards. The difficulties faced in carrying out audit outside a system of clinical audit are related to the fact that, when several professionals all contribute to the care of a patient, it is impossible to distinguish the outcomes of the care each one has given. At what point, therefore, can anyone be said to be accountable?

There has been considerable resistance to clinical audit, mainly from the medical profession, who seem to be nervous about sharing the results of the scrutiny of care with their colleagues. Part of the difficulty has been the original emphasis on medical audit by the government, who thought that in order to encourage the uptake of audit in general it would be necessary to convince the medical profession first. A great deal of money has been spent on medical audit, and it may be hard to now wean the medical profession off the idea that the information gained is for their use only.

In fact, other groups have tended to embrace audit rather more enthusiastically than many doctors, perhaps because of the recognition of its potential for increasing autonomy and accountability. The reluctance to disclose information about practice to colleagues, which is necessary in clinical audit, may also be due to the vulnerability doctors feel about legal proceedings. This assumes that accountability has implications for liability which cannot be avoided, and this in turn raises questions about ownership of care and who the referent others really are.

Surely the patients, who are the paying public, have a right to know that there is a system in place to safeguard their interests? It has too long been the case that professionalism has been equated with freedom to act at will in a context in which a patient was viewed as a case, an example of a disease process or a medical condition. In such a context the patient and their care 'belonged' to the professional, with litigation being the only mechanism available for the patient to bring the professional to account. It is hoped that clinical audit and similar QA techniques will enable a more positive disclosure to take place, with colleagues acting on behalf of the patients as referent others through a system of peer review, and for subsequent improvements to be made to care and hence the need for litigation to be reduced.

The suspicion of clinical audit and nervousness about its employment reflect the discomfort that recounting – as distinct from accounting – can cause, and illustrates the need for caution in the introduction of any QA system as a way of implementing accountability. We should not lose sight of the principle on which practitioner-based audit is based.

The issues of ownership of information and the ownership of outcomes, which discussions about clinical audit raise, have serious implications for how effective QA – and audit in particular – can be in implementing accountability in practice. If a positive outcome ensues, who can take the credit? If, on the other hand, there is a negative outcome, who is at fault? Is it the doctor, the nurse, the paramedic or the domestic? In order for professionals to take personal account of their actions, there needs to be a way for those actions to be noted as discrete, and as having some sort of discernible effect on the patient. It may be that it is not the final outcome – total recovery or death, for example – against which actions are measured, but the intermediate or proximal outcomes, as they are known. The development of clear intermediate outcomes that can be attributed to each professional group, and even to individuals within those groups, becomes an imperative and an added incentive to the development of structured and systematic methods of accountability.

Autonomy

If the model of clinical audit is used, standard setting by professionals offers a structure for deciding the parameters of their autonomy, and hence for what they can be considered accountable. By re-establishing the patient as the ultimate referent other, and by accepting that peer review is an intermediate step between disclosing to the patient in person and a solely external mechanism of regulation, some sense of working together towards a common goal should be achieved. The common goal can be then further refined to give a standard for the achievement of defined criteria sets which delineate the responsibilities of each professional group. By standard setting together in this way, each group is accorded the authority to discharge its responsibility as defined in the standard. Disclosure then takes the form of a demonstration of the results of audit to peers, with the potential for further public scrutiny, if necessary, through either audit committees or service purchasers.

As the responsibilities defined within the standard take account of the codes of conduct for each professional group, there remains an external regulation to further safeguard the interests of the patient. In this way each practitioner can operate autonomously within a team of fellow professionals.

The dynamic standard-setting system has been used successfully for clinical audit in this way in a number of settings, notably postoperative pain management (Cunningham and Hiscock 1992) and the care of people with learning disabilities (Marr and McRae 1992). The success of the approach seems to lie in the fact that all those who take part in the group consider the patient to be the prime referent other, and to feel that everyone involved is equally accountable for the care the patient receives.

Hierarchies are disposed of in the mechanism of the group, where people are encouraged to contribute as equals by the use of a facilitator. The role of the facilitator is very important in the achievement of standards and the sense of equal value that is necessary in all contributors to this task.

THE PITFALLS: CHANGING A CULTURE TO ENABLE CHANGES IN PRACTICE

The sense of equality is one of the key factors in determining whether QA as a mechanism for implementing accountability in nursing will ever be successful.

The practitioner-based approach is limited in fulfilling the criteria for assuming accountability described by Lewis and Batey (1982a,b). The problem seems to be rooted in the question of authority and, in consequence, autonomy.

Nurses attempting to use standard setting as a way of exercising authority in defining goals for care and the methods of achieving them, and to use these standards as a process of putting accountability into operation, still have the problem that their success will be limited by the amount of autonomy they have in the work situation. They often have to work within a culture which is reluctant to give up the power a hierarchical structure affords those in senior positions, or one which is slow to recognize the changes taking place within nursing. This gives rise to an increasingly well educated staff who have the authority of research-based knowledge and skills to assume a level of autonomy and accountability previously unknown.

This reluctance is evidenced by the difficulty some nurses face when trying to implement practitioner-based systems of QA without the fully negotiated and demonstrably committed support of management and other senior staff. The potential for sabotage by the power of veto is immense. A distinction, of course, has to be made between a veto for professional reasons and one made for other reasons.

Although nurses may write their own standards or tailor externally written standards, they currently send them to senior management for both ratification and support. Where the manager's signature represents support for the standard and a concomitant pledge to work towards providing any resources needed to achieve it, this does in some way accord power to the nurses by acknowledging that they have the knowledge to make decisions regarding care and to define their responsibilities in carrying out that care. The nurses are also accorded the power of disclosure, deciding themselves how often to audit the standard, who the auditors will be, and what will be disclosed and to whom. In organizations where managers exercise the power of veto for control, perhaps for budgetary reasons, there is clearly less chance of the standards being used to either exercise or demonstrate the nurses' accountability as professionals.

The question of veto takes us back to the original discussion about responsibility, authority and autonomy. In the drive to make nurses more accountable, it is worth considering the structures and hierarchies of medicine as a profession, so that we do not give too much accountability to people who do not have either the authority or the autonomy to assume certain responsibilities, or to be accountable for their discharge. The power of veto illustrates this. Medical consultants do not supervise junior doctors; instead, they discuss decisions regarding care and only veto decisions which are either erroneous or beyond the scope of the particular junior doctor's authority. This in no way undermines the junior doctor as a professional, and the consultant continues to expect the junior doctor to be personally accountable for all the responsibilities they assume. In nursing, by contrast, the sister or charge nurse is held accountable for all the care carried out by the nursing staff who work on a ward. How does the charge nurse exercise the power of veto in this situation? Are staff nurses held personally accountable for the care they plan, and are junior staff nurses held accountable themselves, to the senior staff nurse, or directly to the sister or charge nurse? To whose standards does the nurse work and do they have to recount what they have done, or is there a planned method for its disclosure?

We have discussed the fact that it is possible to set up a system that affords nurses greater autonomy, and thereby accountability, perhaps based on a model such as primary nursing. Team nursing can also be used to give the power for decision-making back to the individual through the medium of team goal setting and care planning. Supervision can then be carried out, in theory, in a way similar to that of the consultant. The senior nurse can then play the role of ward manager more effectively, exercising the power of veto when there are uncertainties about a planned aspect of care, in a way that does not undermine the professional integrity of the nurse.

Standards, and their audit in the scenario in which they are set and audited by the professionals themselves, can be seen to perform a triple function in promoting internal regulation and the wellbeing of the patient. The first function is that they help the individual nurse to clarify how they intend to act, through the setting of a clear objective. How best to achieve this standard and the effectiveness of the chosen processes is checked by a consideration of the available research and a critical appraisal of the experiences of those setting the standard in developing the criteria sets. Secondly, the standard setting provides an educational function in which more experienced nurses share their knowledge with junior staff. There is evaluation of research findings, and innovations can be generated by the group. Thirdly, the clear definition of the care to be given within the criteria also accords a role to an external auditor, a necessary characteristic if QA is to be used for the purposes of accountability as defined by Lewis and Batey (1982a). They state that within QA the roles and responsibilities of all those involved in an activity should be defined to enable the auditor to ensure that the responsibility is only being carried by someone with the authority to do so.

New knowledge may come from standard setting, but one of the criticisms levelled at the practitioner-based approach reflects a concern with the knowledge, and therefore the authority to act, that nurses currently have. Can standards written by nurses working in the field be said to demonstrate the state of the art in nursing, and can they therefore be used to replace the protocols of experts? Research carried out to evaluate the dynamic standard-setting system suggests that there is a fairly good degree of congruence in the identification of key criteria by nurses working on the ward and those identified by other experts in whatever subject is under scrutiny. This is exemplified by the research into postoperative pain management (RCN 1993b).

If QA and audit are to remain viable as a method for implementing accountability the standards clearly need to include guidelines or criteria which have been evaluated for effectiveness. This, in turn, emphasizes the need for the development of measures of that effectiveness – the outcomes. Both the process of achieving the standards and the anticipated outcomes need to be examined in some detail. A major difficulty in reaching this goal is the multidimensional nature of health care, which was considered above. There is also a need to think of outcomes in a way which is broader than the apparent endpoint of care. Such outcomes – so-called proximal outcomes – are dependent on rigorous research into health care and the application of the findings. A search of the literature is very much to be encouraged when standards are being set. A difficulty arises, however, in that for many subjects in nursing there is a paucity of good research, particularly regarding the outcomes of various clinical practices. Part of the solution to this problem would be to change the current approach to nursing research, which seems at times haphazard and competitive to the point of secrecy, to one in which priorities are made clear by the nurses themselves and which are planned for with a clear strategy for their investigation and the dissemination of findings. This is also a feature of research in other fields of health care, but in nursing it is compounded by the late start nursing has had in educating its practitioners in the techniques and rigours of good scientific enquiry. Hopefully, the recently released strategy for research in nursing, health visiting and midwifery (DoH 1993b) should prove a catalyst to the much-needed research on nursing interventions and their outcomes.

CAN STANDARD SETTING AND AUDIT BE USED TO IMPLEMENT ACCOUNTABILITY IN NURSING?

As a way of achieving accountability QA, through the employment of such as the dynamic standard-setting system, would seem at first glance to be the answer. It gives nurses a means by which to clearly demarcate the areas for which they can legitimately have responsibility, either through setting standards for a nursing topic or by joining with colleagues in clinical audit. By setting their own standards they are able to make decisions about the kind of care that should be employed in a situation, and the way in which it should be carried out. The methods of care they choose to employ can be evaluated for effectiveness, both before being included within the criteria sets of the standards and by the results of audit. Expected outcomes can be clearly defined and written in a way which is measurable. The findings of the most up-to-date research can be included and the standards continually revised to ensure that they represent state-of-the-art practice.

The process of setting the standards, and their audit, promotes internal regulation, with nurses themselves controlling the exercise and the disclosure they wish to make, but it does not abandon the need for some complementary form of external regulation through the public accessibility of such standards and their audit results. Such standards even provide a potential role for the patients, not just as commentators but as active participants in the standard-setting and audit process, thereby activating their position as referent others. In short, standard setting seems to provide both the education and the mechanism for accountability in nursing. Here the chapter should end and you should feel able to go forth and spread the message that accountability is something for nurses to embrace through the medium of QA, but unfortunately it is not quite that simple.

Although it is tempting to equate accountability with the evaluative aspects of QA, in which there is a drive to demonstrate the effectiveness and efficiency of a particular professional's contribution to care, not all writers in the field would view them as one and the same thing, or even elements of one objective. This seems to be partly the result of an association of QA with organizational control and its attendant feature of sanctions. There are also disagreements over definitions of accountability and evaluation. Robinson (1971), for example, claimed that programme accountability deals with both the quality of the work carried out and the determination of whether the programme met the goals set for it. Passos (1973) merged accountability with structures of control by linking it with evaluation; she claimed that accountability was actually a form of evaluation. For Hartnett (1971) evaluation is concerned with effectiveness, whereas accountability focuses on both effectiveness and efficiency. Friedson (1974), concerned about the danger of confusing the positive potential of QA techniques as methods of accountability with the power to bring about change, with their more negative implications involving sanctions, suggested that it is important to constrain an emphasis on sanctioning with professionals and rather to emphasize a self-governing or occupational principle. This highlights the value of QA methods that make a distinction between control and the identification of opportunity for change. Lewis and Batey (1982a,b) confirm that formal disclosure should take place so that decisions can be made, information exchanged and evaluations and sanctions applied, but the application of sanctions is not accountability itself. The response of organizational control structures – the application of formal sanctions – is an organizational reaction to that which is disclosed or not disclosed.

It seems, therefore, that before any decision can be made about whether QA can be used as a method of implementing accountability, we need to be very clear about what we mean by QA and the techniques we are thinking of in particular. Looking at the differing opinions about QA outlined above, it can be seen that they reflect the two main schools of thought regarding QA in nursing: the traditional view of quality through the removal of poor performers, or the practitioner-based approach in which quality is seen as the consequence of capitalizing on identified opportunities for improvement, discovered by the professionals themselves. Clearly, if we subscribe to the latter view then practitioner-based QA is an appropriate mechanism for implementing accountability in nursing. If, instead, we agree with the traditional view of QA as a mechanism for control, it has more in common with mechanisms for external regulation and will do very little to foster any sense of responsibility, authority, autonomy, and hence accountability.

The question of referent others also remains a problem. The patient is often supposed to be the prime referent other, but this is not the reality of the situation in that there are few well established mechanisms to enable this to happen. Often in QA patients are used as contributors to audit data, but only to the extent of providing information. They are often called upon to fill in question-naires or to take part in interviews. This is all felt to legitimate involvement of the community in line with the dictates of the Patient's Charter (DoH 1992a). The problem is, however, that it is very rare for patients to receive feedback about the results of the audit in which they took part, or to discover what changes have been made as a consequence. Even if disclosure were made, what information and help do the patients have in interpreting the facts and figures? What implications do disclosures have on a population whose confidence in the health service providers has been seriously dented in recent years? Even more to the point, however, is that if they are supposed to be the prime referent others, but professional accountability precludes them from having any influ-ence at all on the disclosure agenda, what does this role even mean, and what does this in turn suggest about the favouring of professional accountability to the exclusion of external mechanisms of accounting? Are we pursuing profes-sionalism to the detriment of human rights?

Luckily, for most of us, each regional health authority has bodies established to protect the patient's position as referent other in the form of the Community Health Councils. Other organizations also exist, such as the College of Health and the Patients' Association, whose remit is to promote the interests of patients, but still the question remains, what mechanisms are in place to enable disclosure to take place about the activities of professionals to patients, or at least their representatives?

One method currently being developed is the contracting process between providers and purchasers of the service. The purchasers insist on audit activities being carried out and stipulate a series of targets to be reached for the popula-tion they represent. The difficulty is, of course, that the achievement of targets is a return to a control-type external regulatory mechanism, and it may be quite detached from the needs of a population who may be more concerned with the kind of maintenance of their dignity that someone who feels personally account-able for their care may be able to provide. Another difficulty is the very act of representation. Whether we like it or not, everyone has their own perception of a situation or the needs of a particular population.

Various projects have been set up to investigate whether patients can be involved in both standard setting and in the process of audit and disclosure. Perhaps what we are striving for is a such an internalization of the concept of accountability that every professional, whether nurse, doctor, or paramedic, understands their accountability to the patient in personal terms. It could, in fact, be seen as accountability to ourselves as potential patients. Various texts have been written from this psychological viewpoint, and a more comprehensive discussion of the issues is clearly beyond the scope of this chapter. The important message is, however, to understand that for nurses to achieve accountability in their practice three levels of regulation have to be included. The first is the internal regulation of professional practice, having sufficient authority and autonomy to make decisions about the discharge of legitimate responsibilities, and making self-controlled disclosures about the discharge of these responsibilities to referent others. The second is external regulation, through the power of veto and by the maintenance of powers of licence to practise which protect the public good; and the third is the internalization of the emotional and psychological aspects of accountability. This involves commitment and the ability to appreciate actions and intentions from the referent other's point of view.

CONCLUSION

It is clear that for a move to internal or personal accountability to be achievable for nurses, clearer links between discrete interventions and particular patient outcomes are needed which reflect current research-based knowledge. From these, goals and standards can be set to bridge the gap between external and internal mechanisms of accountability which afford nurses the authority to assume the autonomous role their development as a profession demands.

Demonstrable standards, with attendant audit results, and the evidence of action to remedy any shortfall, also serve as a mechanism by which external regulators acting on behalf of the public can monitor, and if necessary apply sanctions against, the professionals. External mechanisms of accountability such as the UKCC will continue to legitimate the existence of internal mechanisms of accountability by confirming professional status and the authority to assume responsibilities within the parameters of the profession.

Techniques of QA, and in particular standard setting using the practitioner-based approach, can make a valuable contribution to operationalizing the concept of accountability. This gives an analytical and structured approach to the activation of concepts of responsibility, authority and autonomy, as well as the process of disclosure and evaluation. The exercise of standard setting and audit may also contribute to the development of people and a consequently increased willingness, based on experience of taking responsibility for quality, to move professionally to a place of personal accountability.

There is no way that nurses can avoid this challenge. A commitment to focusing care more firmly on the patient already exists. This is exemplified by the development of primary nursing, the inclusion of patients in audit activities, the recognition of the need for more holistic care, and its enshrinement in the Patients' Charter. Focusing on the patient in this way demands that professionals embrace the need for personal accountability, which is, after all, the foundation on which the public's trust in the professions serving them is based. Accountability for the patient as the referent other can therefore be understood as a human right, and as such should be demonstrated in a way that is understandable to all.

5 | Accountability in primary nursing

Sheila Rodgers

INTRODUCTION

Accountability is discussed in this chapter as it relates to primary nursing. An outline of primary nursing will be given so that the reader can appreciate the debates on the matter, and other articles and texts can be consulted for further information (F. Black 1992; Ersser and Tutton 1991; Manthey 1992; Pearson 1988). Similarly, definitions of accountability are not dwelt upon but are discussed in relation to primary nursing.

The chapter begins by introducing some of the key concepts in primary nursing and looks at some of the reasons for its emergence. A more detailed discussion follows, with a specific focus on the issue of accountability. Finally, some conclusions are drawn and a consideration of developments beyond primary nursing is made.

Bergman (1981) states that in order for a person to be held accountable, all of the following are required:

- Ability: the relevant knowledge, skills and values to make decisions and act;
- Responsibility: given to the person to enable them to carry out the action;
- Authority: the formal backing to carry the action through, i.e. the power to make sure that it happens.

Acceptance of responsibility is only one part of accountability: the nurse must also have a relevant balance of ability and authority in order to be held accountable. Responsibility can be delegated for specific tasks which one then has a duty to perform. It is not possible to delegate accountability, as this is more to do with an overall concern for nursing care. The performance of care is then judged by peers, employers and patients against professional standards.

Goulding and Hunt (1991) argue that, until recently, accountability in nursing has been unclear. Nurses may also have felt uncomfortable and sometimes appear overly concerned with the issue of accountability. Accountability is tackled 'head-on' within primary nursing, which has developed clear lines of accountability:

'What primary nursing has done is to take the concept of accountability and be proactive with it, grasping it with enthusiasm' (Evans 1993).

In a hierarchical system, such as the health service and large hospitals, there is usually also a hierarchy of responsibility, therefore different levels of accountability exist. Regardless of their level within the hierarchy, all nurses are held accountable, primarily to the patient, for their sphere of responsibility within the health service. Providing a service to a group of patients, no matter how large, does not diffuse accountability. Managers must still be able to demonstrate that they are acting in the individual patient's best interests – 'to promote and safeguard the wellbeing and interests of the patient' (UKCC 1992a). This might not always be easy to achieve in view of the priorities and demands made by increasing market forces and organizational drives for cost containment and greater efficiency. Whether such organizational aims are compatible with the patients' best interests and wellbeing is a thorny political and moral question which is beyond the remit of this chapter. However, such dilemmas increasingly impinge on the accountability of nurses for an individual patient's care.

Manthey (1992) suggests that primary nursing is a way of giving professional care within a bureaucratic structure. Bureaucracies tend to consist of groups, with decisions being made by the group's head. Care is provided according to routine and procedure, with the objectives being to meet organizational aims such as high throughput and smooth running of the group. Primary nursing aims to minimize bureaucracy and make hospital care more individualized. Primary nursing depends on a flattened hierarchical structure so that nurses can have autonomy and authority over patient care.

Primary nursing is not, however, an end in itself but one way of achieving individualized and humanistic care provided by accountable nurses. It is not necessarily the only way in which to achieve these goals, nor does it solve the problems of under-resourcing or increased workloads. It has been argued that primary nursing may be more cost-effective in eliminating unnecessary routinized care and providing care according to individual need (Manthey 1992). Primary nursing is a system of delivering care that enables or empowers nurses to reach their full potential in caring for their patients. It therefore facilitates high-quality care but does not necessarily ensure it. Primary nursing offers an opportunity for nursing to become patient centred and to realize congruence between education and practice (Wright 1991). There is evidence of improved staff morale and patient satisfaction in primary nursing, as staff recruitment and retention is improved and turnover falls (Alexander *et al.* 1981; Blair *et al.* 1982; Bond *et al.* 1991). Staff therefore work more efficiently, and Wright

(1991) argues that this, and the increase in expertise, outweighs the costs of the rises in staff increments.

THE RISING POPULARITY OF PRIMARY NURSING

Educationists in nursing are currently striving for professionalization through the introduction of the 1992 programmes of education which were first introduced in demonstration districts in 1989 (Project 2000). However, nursing practice in many areas has not itself been professionalized (Manthey 1992). There is little autonomy in decision-making, performance review is carried out by superiors rather than peers, and it is usually seen as being potentially punitive. The abilities and potential of nurses are not being realized.

In team or task nursing, the registered nurse or the highest-qualified nurse does the technical, highest-status tasks and supervises the other less-qualified nurses (Pearson and Vaughan 1986). Manthey (1992) describes task and team nursing in the following way:

> 'Registered nurses in these systems are not professional caregivers, rather they are checker uppers of cheaper doers.'

The increasing popularity of primary nursing may, in part, be due to a dissatisfaction with this. Although team and task nursing are nominally two different delivery systems, team nursing can often revert to mini-task allocation. Nurses are graded by skills and there is fragmentation of care. There may be patient allocation within team nursing but care is still directed by the team leader and not by the caregivers. There may also be a lack of continuity as different nurses care for different patients each day. Perhaps one of the major criticisms of team nursing is that channels of communication are complex and potentially confusing. Information may be passed from caregiver to team leader, to charge nurse, to external agency (such as medical staff), and back again through the hierarchy. In such a system an inordinate amount of time is spent on communication, which becomes diluted and sometimes distorted.

Lack of accountability in team nursing

Another major criticism of team nursing is the shared responsibility and the lack of accountability. The team leader makes the decisions about patient care and devolves the responsibility for delivering it to the direct caregiver. The responsibility for care is thereby split. Where there is no patient allocation within teams, responsibility may be even further diffused. Sharing responsibility in these situations makes lines of accountability unclear or, as Manthey (1992) says, 'Shared responsibility equals no responsibility'.

Within team nursing care plans may not be completed or updated because the shared responsibility for doing so means that it is no one person's responsibility. Teams may also tend to function without care plans, as the care contin-ues to be routinized and bureaucratic rather than individualized. The role of the team leader takes the most highly qualified nurse in each team away from direct caregiving. Team leaders allocate themselves as few as possible of the less dependent patients so that they can fulfil the high-status technical tasks and supervise other nurses. The most highly qualified nurse, therefore, gives little direct care. This is not to say that the role of team leader is an easy one – they have to plan care based on the assessments and evaluations of other less-qualified nurses, and retain full information about all patients in order to report back on them.

It has already been argued that care plans and the nursing process are redun-dant in a bureaucratic, routinized system of care. The increasing popularity of primary nursing is almost inevitable if the nursing process is to be truly imple-mented, as it is one real way of making the nursing process workable (Bowers 1989).

Visibility and responsibility

Nurses working in such a system might feel threatened by their anticipated exposure to increased accountability in primary nursing. However, direct visi-bility, personal responsibility and increased accountability have been suggested as some of the very reasons for the popularity of primary nursing. Bowers (1989) states:

'Current popularity in the United Kingdom may well be linked to the current vogue for clearly delineated (on paper) lines of responsibility, with accountability passed down from the centre to those on the front line of the service.'

The needs of nurses striving for professionalism in practice may also be met through primary nursing. The role of the nurse is defined in bedside care rather than through managerial structures, and there is increasing autonomy for prac-tice and a freedom from medical and hierarchical dominance. Increasing profes-sionalism thus enables nurses to control nursing and to share this autonomy with patients.

Initiatives such as the named nurse have further epitomized demands for lines of responsibility and accountability. Some have seen named nursing as having many similarities with primary nursing. However, primary nursing, it has been consistently argued, is a bottom-up change requiring full commitment from the ward staff to the change in roles and practices. Primary nursing cannot be successfully imposed by managers (Johns 1991).

Despite the arguments of professionalism, consumerism and social and legislative demands for the development of primary nursing, the supporting evidence regarding patient outcomes is scant. Much research in primary nursing is small scale, lacking in methodological rigour, and does not adequately operationally define primary nursing. (Recent research has developed a tool to evaluate definitions of primary nursing – Mead 1991). Many early studies on primary nursing focused upon nurse or patient satisfaction and not on the patient's health outcome. Research on systems of care and assessing patient outcome is complex and demanding. However, it would seem essential to pursue such research rather than a partially sighted acceleration towards an unknown goal. McCormack (1991) and F. Black (1992) both give extensive reviews of research in primary nursing.

PRIMARY NURSING AS A PROFESSIONAL PRACTICE DELIVERY SYSTEM

The movement towards increasing accountability and responsibility, giving increasing control of individual actions, allows nursing to move further towards a professional practice delivery system. Three key elements to such a system have been identified:

- the clear allocation and acceptance of responsibility for decision making;
- the delegation to an individual of authority which is commensurate with ability;
- the establishment of mechanisms of accountability so that the quality of the decisions that have been made can be evaluated (Manthey 1992).

A further feature of professional practice delivery systems might be standard setting and review by peers, leading to further professional practice development. Clearly, accountability is central to such a system. Primary nursing can be seen as one way of achieving professional practice, and has been defined as:

'The delivery of comprehensive, coordinated, continuous and individualized patient care through the professional nurse who has autonomy, accountability and authority. There is an allocation and acceptance of 24 hour, 7 days a week individual responsibility for nursing care to one named nurse, with the care planner as caregiver' (Manthey 1980).

Continuity of care

Continuity of care is implied as being from admission to discharge, and may also include readmission. The responsibility for patient care is continuously with the primary nurse, from whom there is direct communication with the associate nurse and all others involved in the patient's care. The primary nurse relies on detailed care plans for associate nurses to follow in their absence. Such plans are essential, as care is individualized and does not follow routines or procedures.

The care planner as caregiver is an important concept that brings the primary nurse to the bedside in order to assess and evaluate care. The primary nurse has autonomy and, thereby, the freedom to make decisions and act upon them. Authority is invested in the primary nurses by the charge nurse, giving them the power to act and make decisions.

The three key concepts of responsibility, authority and autonomy are well defined in primary nursing. Goulding and Hunt (1991) outline them as follows:

- Responsibility: a charge for which one is answerable. The focus is on the charge, not on how or to whom the answering should occur;
- Authority: the rightful (legitimate) power to fulfil a charge (responsibility). Authority in nursing derives from at least three sources: authority of the situation; authority of expert knowledge; authority of position;
- Autonomy: a means of self-determination, self-direction, freedom to design a total plan of nursing care and to work on an independent level with other professionals; being left on one's own to work.

Primary nurses may delegate responsibility to their associates in their absence. Both must ensure that nurses to whom responsibilities are delegated first accept those responsibilities, secondly have the competence to carry them out, and thirdly, acknowledge limitations in their competence, refusing to accept such responsibilities without having received instruction and been assessed as competent. In this respect, autonomy is bound by the limits of the nurse's own knowledge, skill, experience and authority.

Accountability in primary nursing is continuous from admission to discharge. In patient allocation, continuity may be for the duration of a span of duty. In team nursing it may be for a group of patients by a group of nurses. In task allocation, by contrast, accountability rests solely with the charge nurse.

Continuous accountability allows for the long-term effects of nursing care to be evaluated, and also facilitates consistency of care. The situation is hopefully avoided where one nurse decides on one day that a patient should shower and dress, while another, on the next day, feels that the patient should be washed in bed and not dressed, despite no apparent change in condition. It is not that such confusions cannot be resolved by other means, but the system of care delivery in primary nursing can serve to prevent such problems. Resorting to blanket ward policies and procedures is of little or no benefit to individual patients. Nor can any nurse be held truly accountable for care, apart from the one setting the procedures and policies. If this is shared, then responsibility becomes diffuse and ineffective.

In order to become an autonomous, accountable practitioner the primary nurse must have commensurate abilities, including an extensive knowledge base and the ability to learn from and reflect upon situations. Nursing decisions and actions must be derived from these abilities. Decisions about a patient's care are made by one nurse, from admission to discharge, therefore it is clear who is accountable. This enables a shift towards patient-centred care rather than the emphasis being on routinization with the primary function of serving organizational goals rather than those of individual need.

Primary nursing also demands clarification of the boundaries of responsibility. In the past:

'...they (nurses) have not been directly accountable for individual patient care before, have not been generally held to account for their work and have had limited access to their personal capabilities' (Johns 1990).

What are nurses responsible for?

Nurses have often been unsure what they are responsible for and what they have authority over. They also need to be sure of their own personal capabilities, i.e. what they **can** be responsible for. Previously this has not been questioned, as nurses were constrained by bureaucracy, hierarchy and limited autonomy. However, if these constraints are to be removed, one must be sure of personal boundaries (Johns 1990).

If nurses are forced to accept responsibility for work beyond their personal capabilities, then not only is this potentially disastrous for the patient, but nurses will react defensively to protect themselves from anxiety. The role of primary nurse must not be imposed on those who are unable to draw on adequate personal capabilities of knowledge, experience and reflection on practice. Managers must be aware that primary nursing and the role of primary nurse cannot be imposed for this very reason, among others. An imbalance in any of the elements of ability, autonomy and authority will prevent the development of a professional practice delivery system such as primary nursing.

Education and preparation

A high level of educational preparation is required for primary nursing in order to prepare nurses for increased demands on their abilities, greater visibility and the increased requirements of accountability and decision-making. The sense of responsibility involved in becoming a primary nurse should not be underestimated. Some nurses may need extensive preparation, including education, further experience and decision-making and communication skills. A high level of competence is required if the primary nurse is to plan, direct and deliver patient care independently, without deferring decisions to the charge nurse. Any improvements in quality of care are highly dependent on preparation and continued development.

'The quality of care depends upon the quality of the primary nurse. Merely allocating nurses to patients is no guarantee that care will get better' (Wright 1991).

Patient allocation, or the case method, is only one element of the structure of primary nursing (Figure 5.1). In a study of nurses working with primary nursing McCormack (1991) found that higher levels of stress were experienced by the more junior staff nurses than by the primary nurses with more experience. The importance of education, experience and preparation was thought to be significant. When the numbers of registered nurses on duty fell and the skill mix became poorer, the staff nurses felt an increased responsibility for all patients on the ward plus the supervision of students and nursing assistants. This proved to be a source of much strain and anxiety. Such a situation is not created by primary nursing, the skill mix workload being independent of the delivery system. However, primary nursing served to highlight the issues of accountability and responsibility which made the nurses more aware of the problems and led to anxiety.

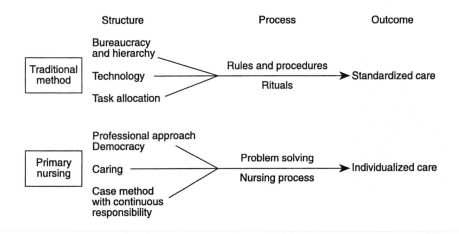

Figure 5.1 The system of primary nursing compared to the traditional method. (Source: Binnie 1990)

McCormack (1991) also found that nurses working in primary nursing had highly developed values and concepts of nursing, but used the terms accountability and responsibility interchangeably. Associate nurses (who carried out prescribed care in the primary nurses' absence) felt a duty in performing specific tasks, whereas primary nurses were more concerned with the overall care of the patient. The nurses felt they had more autonomy in primary nursing than in other more traditional staff nurse posts, but were frustrated by constraints on their autonomy, such as bureaucratic management.

The role of the charge nurse

The role of the charge nurse in primary nursing is crucial. The prime function of the charge nurse is to manage the ward so that the registered nurses can manage patient care. The charge nurse is responsible for ensuring that the primary nurses are fully equipped (educationally, in terms of knowledge and skills) and supported so that they can be responsible and accountable for the care they prescribe. The charge nurse remains accountable for, and becomes more actively involved with, the quality and standards of care on the ward. Thereby, in a system of primary nursing they become more truly accountable for the ward. The charge nurse is seen as a leader, facilitator, change agent, manager, educator and clinical expert (Table 5.1). The charge nurse has a key role to play in managing the ward while promoting professional practice.

Table 5.1 The role of the charge nurse

Clinical expert	gives advice and training
Resource	for nurses and staff supporter
Facilitator	assisting nurses to develop knowledge and skills
Teacher	prepares primary nurses to a level of ability so that they can accept their own patients
Monitor	of standards and quality of care and individual care plans
Manager	of ward staff, employment procedures, resources, staff rostering, budgeting, accounting etc.
Manager	of quality assurance programmes
Associate nurse	may act as an associate nurse in teaching by role modelling and in evaluating care plans
Primary nurse	may act as a primary nurse for a small caseload of patients on occasions, in order to act as a role model and continue to develop her own expertise

A bureaucratic organization sets policies and procedures that will ensure the smooth running of the organization and control large numbers of staff. The organization puts itself first, whereas the professional puts individual patients' needs first. Professional practice within such a system can be severely limited unless the charge nurse is able to absorb such pressures at ward management level.

'The task is to manage the gap between the needs of the organization and the demands of professional practice for autonomy' (Johns 1990).

In order for the charge nurse to begin to meet such a demanding task, the necessary authority, autonomy and responsibility must be devolved to their level. The charge nurse must be able to control the ward budget, ward policies, staffing and recruitment, for instance. Managers contemplating imposing a primary nursing system will find a conflict of philosophy here, and must be prepared to devolve such responsibility and authority and move away from hierarchical, bureaucratic management styles. The commitment required should not be underestimated. Johns (1990) remains pessimistic:

'In a world dominated by budget constraints and an increasing trained staff shortage, the organization is likely to maintain a pragmatic approach to organizing care rather than pursuing an ideological approach irrespective of its humanity attraction.'

Perhaps this can be seen to support the need to strive for increasing professionalization within nursing in order to humanize hospital care in a climate dominated by costs rather than value.

Relations with medical staff

Frustration in relations with medical staff has also been reported in primary nursing (Roberts 1980). This may be due to the increasing professionalization of nursing, leading to a power struggle as nurses attempt to define the boundaries of nursing (limits of responsibility) and function independently. Along with educational development and an increase in depth of knowledge regarding individual patient care, nurses no longer play the doctor/nurse game. McCormack (1991) quotes a nurse in primary nursing talking about medical staff relationships:

'...they almost feel threatened by the knowledge you have of the patients and they don't want to make it seem like you are making the decision.'

Undoubtedly some medical staff also find adjusting to working with primary nurses stressful as they encounter new sets of values and have their boundaries challenged.

The UKCC (United Kingdom Central Council for Nursing, Midwifery and Health Visiting) code of conduct (UKCC 1992a) clause on collaboration applies not only to relationships with medical and other health-care staff but also to other primary and associate nurses. Primary nurses may work consistently with the same group of associate nurses and nursing assistants caring for the same group of patients, and so may work in isolation – apart from monitoring from the charge nurse. Primary nurses have a responsibility to support each other and share information and knowledge. Collaboration and peer review are essential, otherwise primary nurses may simply develop 'mini routines' or 'mini policies', routinely selecting nursing actions that they personally have become most familiar with and in which they have faith. Primary nurses must open themselves to challenge and debate and demonstrate accountability to their peers. This can be extremely powerful and defensive responses to feedback may occur if nurses work outside their personal capabilities. If this is the case it should be recognized as such, and the need for further development and support acknowledged.

Primary nursing could also lead to primary nurses and teams working competitively. McCormack (1991) found that nurses developed close relationships with their group of patients and felt a true sense of responsibility and ownership. However, this did make ending relationships difficult, and ownership progressed to possessiveness. Primary and associate nurses caring for the same group of patients leads to continuity of care, but McCormack also found that some nurses became unwilling to care for the patients of other primary nursing teams. If one accepts the argument that continuity of care is maintained by the primary nurse's care plan, then the necessity for associate nurses and nursing assistants to work with the same group of patients no longer holds. It may reduce possessiveness and competitiveness and create flexibility if associates and nursing assistants maintain a working knowledge of all patients in the ward by having patients assigned daily.

In some models of primary nursing, all experienced staff nurses work as primary nurses with a small group of patients while acting as associates for each other. Manthey (1991) has advocated such a model for reducing inter-team conflict and reducing the size of the caseload for each. It also eliminates any hierarchy created by different levels of responsibility.

Decentralization of decision-making

One of the founding principles of primary nursing is decentralized decision-making and the elimination of hierarchical structures. However, the charge nurse, primary nurse and associate nurse all have different levels of responsibility, autonomy and accountability. The primary nurse retains overall responsibility and is held accountable for the patients' care throughout their stay in the ward. This is only possible if the primary nurses' decisions and plans are carried through in their absence. They must have the authority to prescribe care throughout the patient's stay, and this implies authority over associate nurses. Evans (1993) has suggested that this should mean the primary nurse being the line manager of the associate nurse, being involved in recruitment and appraisal. F. Black (1992) argues that such an approach creates a new hierarchy that undermines the principles of primary nursing. It could be argued that authority has not only to be legitimate (conferred by the institution) but, perhaps more importantly in primary nursing, mutually agreed by colleagues. This could happen by virtue of a primary nurse's close personal knowledge of an individual patient and acknowledged expertise and ability in managing that patient's care.

The authority of the primary nurse is agreed and not challenged unless there are unforeseen changes in a patient's condition. Changes in care may then be made by an associate nurse, usually in consultation with another primary nurse or the charge nurse. These changes must be justified when the primary nurse returns to duty, the associate thereby being held to account for their own decisions and actions. (In some cases primary nurses have agreed to be called at home in order to make changes to a patient's care plan, but this approach has not been widely accepted in the UK.) Associate nurses may find having to make decisions about changes to a primary nurse's care plan stressful and filled with uncertainty. Discussions with colleagues can resolve some of this, but it is almost inevitable as nursing decisions are rarely made with full information (Manthey 1992).

In a collegial system (i.e. when primary nurses also work as associates and primary nurse teams do not exist) the requirement for direct line management over associate nurses is not necessary. Hierarchy and bureaucracy are thus limited.

Health-care assistants

The role of nursing assistants or health-care assistants (HCA) in primary nursing has been widely debated. The issue of untrained assistants caring for patients exists outwith primary nursing, but primary nursing forces nurses to address the issue head on. Nursing students are, on the whole, no longer part of the workforce, but may deliver nursing care under the supervision of a registered nurse in order to meet learning needs. The withdrawal of students from the workforce has undoubtedly led to an increase in the use of HCAs, and their contribution to primary nursing requires clarification.

One suggestion, which appears quite idealistic, is that HCAs assist nurses in their work, are assigned to nurses and not to patients, and perform non-nursing duties. The reality of most situations is that HCAs are assigned to so-called 'basic' nursing tasks. Fragmentation thus occurs and fundamental aspects of nursing care are devalued.

Holistic care

Primary nursing values a holistic approach to care and would discount the existence of 'basic' care. Regardless of the level of technical skill involved, it is the integration of knowledge, critical analysis of data, teaching and comforting skills that humanizes care within hospitals and establishes therapeutic relationships. Assistants may be taught 'complex' technical skills such as blood pressure recording and dressing changes, and supposedly simple tasks such as bed-bathing and feeding patients. However, it is the patient assessment during the process and the interpretation of such an assessment utilizing an extensive knowledge base and personal experience, and expressing appropriate aspects of caring, that leads to a therapeutic relationship. This cannot be done by technicians or assistants, but only by nurses. Primary nursing embraces the support of nursing assistants but also values the central importance of the care planner as caregiver. The primary nurse must deliver sufficient care to evaluate its impact and make decisions regarding further care.

If primary nursing upholds the value of holistic care and refutes task assignment as fragmenting care, how can nursing assistants contribute within this system? Manthey (1991) suggests that HCAs work in a partnership with registered nurses, taking the same shifts and working with the same caseload of patients. The HCA is well known to the registered nurse and a strong working relationship is established. Decisions about who carries out which aspects of care are based on patient need and not tasks. It may be more appropriate for the registered nurse to care for a patient's basic hygiene when they have complex needs (e.g. support regarding body image changes). The nursing assistant may care for the patient with more technical needs, and may require further training to carry out such tasks. However, evaluation and interpretation remain with the registered nurse, who is therefore accountable for the care of all patients in their group. Manthey (1991) also advocates this form of partnership as a method of preceptorship with newly registered nurses.

Other advantages of the partnership system are that primary nurses may take care of their own patients and also act as associates caring for a further group of patients. They are responsible for seeing that the care is given to their associate patients according to their primary nurse's care plan, and are accountable for their own actions but not the overall plan of care. The primary nurse can therefore care for a larger group of patients and directly supervise the work of the HCA or newly qualified nurse, giving one-to-one responsibility (Figure 5.2).

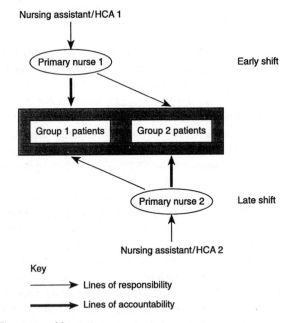

Figure 5.2 The partnership system.

Where primary nurses also work as associates they expose themselves to peer review as their peers attempt to follow their care plans. Also, patients' access to a variety of highly skilled nurses is assured. One criticism of primary nursing has been that patients may not have equal access to the whole team of nurses on the ward. Skill differences between staff tend to be denied, as they are thought to disrupt the team and to introduce status and hierarchy, but it would seem unreasonable not to acknowledge nurses' expertise in different areas and allocate patients accordingly. Nurses should also be encouraged to share knowledge and experience and criticize each other's care (peer accountability), thereby enabling all nurses to develop and extend their personal capabilities.

It may also be argued that, although some primary nurses are more highly skilled than others, this is less important than the continuity, individual relationships and plan of care that are established through primary nursing. Nurses are also challenged to acknowledge their own limitations and capabilities, and should be more aware of when advice or further knowledge from a colleague is required.

Patient autonomy

The autonomy of the nurse in primary nursing can be seen to be increased but does this detract from patient autonomy? The patient does not have free choice on admission as to who will be their primary nurse. Even if choice were offered, the patient would have little knowledge and no experience of the nurses on which to base any judgement. Patients being readmitted may be in a better position here, but this introduces the possibility of unfair discrimination. It should be possible for a patient to change primary nurses during their stay if there is sufficient reason and a strong desire. Such a change need not be negative, but may be due to natural relationships forming when a patient has received more care from another primary nurse working as an associate, or when a nurse has cared for the patient during a critical or significant incident that has left him/her closely involved with that patient's care. Such 'natural selection' does occur and should be acknowledged. The patient may also develop special needs, which may be best served by another primary nurse with the particular expertise required.

In primary nursing the patients may be more autonomous as they can be involved in planning individualized care with their primary nurse. However, McCormack (1991) found that patient autonomy was not always easy to achieve. In high-turnover surgery the patients were involved in the nursing handover but it was more difficult to involve them in care planning owing to the pressure of work and the routine nature of some of the surgery. One nurse reported that she thought the nurse decided what the patient's needs were rather than the patient. Also, as the nurses worked closely with a small group of patients they knew their care plan well and tended to hold it in their heads rather than writing it down. If nurses fail to inform, educate and plan care mutually with patients then they are failing in accountability to the patient.

The power that primary nurses may derive from an in-depth knowledge of all aspects of a patient's care may be potentially threatening both to other professionals and to the patients. However, Leach (1993) found that nurses did not overtly exercise this power and were perhaps unaware of its potential in determining the health care of their patients. Primary nurses may develop a role as 'gatekeeper' as they become pivotal negotiators in patient care, and must be aware of the implications of this.

Nevertheless, a comparison of nurses' autonomy with that of other health-care professionals would not seem to support such a development. Physiotherapists, occupational therapists, medical social workers and speech therapists all have similar educational backgrounds to nurses but differ in being able to work autonomously – to make decisions about care, to make referrals, to operate their own clinics, and to take direct/self-referrals. Nurses still work almost exclusively under medical control, where doctors make referrals, admission, discharges and treatments. The unique function of the nurse is still unclear. At worst it could be seen as 'servicing beds' in order for doctors to treat their patients. Primary nursing aims to help nurses to define nursing and also to define the boundaries of autonomous professional practice.

ACCOUNTABILITY IN PRIMARY NURSING

Lewis and Batey (1982a,b) define accountability as 'a formal obligation to disclose aspects of performance for which the nurse has authority'. The bodies to whom these disclosures should be made are manifold. This has been termed pluralistic accountability (Table 5.2).

Table 5.2 Pluralistic accountability in primary nursing

The primary nurse is accountable to:	
The organization –	to fulfil the job description
The patient –	for outcomes of care
Oneself –	for giving care to the best of one's ability (which only oneself can determine) and for continued knowledge and skill development
Peers –	to support and share with each other knowledge and information on patient care, judging care against agreed standards and the appropriateness of care
The profession –	for the UKCC code of conduct

Not only is accountability pluralistic, it can vary with the level of the nurse in the organization or hierarchy. In a traditional system, authority is retained within the higher levels of the hierarchy and the organization therefore tends to accept vicarious liability for its employees. Delegation of authority has previously stopped at charge nurse level, therefore it has often been the charge nurse who has been held to account for nursing care within a ward. The UKCC code of conduct (UKCC 1992a), however, clearly states that individual nurses are accountable for their own practice. This remains a source of confusion. Many

aspects of care are undertaken by second level nurses, student nurses and n
ing assistants. It is, therefore, quite difficult in a traditional system to ident.
who is accountable for the care of a particular patient and for any omissions c
care.

In primary nursing, it is the primary nurses who have ultimate control over
their patients' care. They may seek advice but it is they who make the final
decision about the plan of care and who are therefore ultimately accountable. In
the traditional system accountability is often diffused and is therefore difficult
to put into operation. The final accountability is supposed to be with the charge
nurse, but different levels of responsibility, and delegated and perceived authority, exist in the hierarchy associated with terms such as 'in charge', 'senior
nurse on duty' and 'team leader'.

Who is accountable?

Tingle (1992c) has challenged the ultimate accountability of the primary nurse,
arguing that the charge nurse remains legally accountable for the primary nurse
in a ward and must therefore supervise him/her and countermand care plans
prescribed by a primary nurse. The circumstances would seem to be exceptional
in which countermanding or intervention may be required. Tingle goes on to
clarify such circumstances as being when the charge nurse 'was convinced that
care was wrong and going to harm the patient'. Surely it is the duty of every
nurse to challenge care which they believe is wrong and potentially harmful?

The primary nurse is accountable to the charge nurse by disclosing aspects of
performance for which he/she has authority. If the charge nurse was required to
countermand plans of care, or frequently challenged the primary nurse, the
authority of that nurse would be undermined and he/she could then only be held
responsible for delegated care, not accountable.

The relationship of the charge nurse to the primary nurse must be one of
teacher, supporter, guide and facilitator. When the charge nurse decides that a
nurse has the ability to work as a primary nurse, authority for patient care is
given to that nurse. This implies that ultimate control and accountability rest
with the manager who delegates.

'Authority, with ensuing autonomy for action, are prerequisites to holding
the primary nurse accountable for the action she takes' (Johns 1990).

The charge nurse should rarely challenge a primary nurse's plan of care but
would expect the primary nurses to justify their actions, explore alternatives
with them and arrive at mutual decisions. In this way the expertise of the
primary nurse is developed and the charge nurse is able to monitor standards of
care. In the collegial climate of primary nursing, peer review is often used as a
powerful means of evaluating standards of care. Such disclosure to peers is not
only an expression of professional accountability but also another opportunity
to share knowledge and understanding, in order that a patient's care has input

from a wider range of expertise, and serves to protect patients from poor-quality practices. Case or team meetings, which are now a common feature of primary nursing, exist in part to serve this function. Being held to account, then, is no longer seen as a defensive experience but as a non-threatening learning experience.

Dealing with mistakes

Nursing has traditionally been intolerant of human fallibility (Manthey 1992) and usually deals with mistakes, errors or omissions through punishment. Primary nursing requires a supportive collegial atmosphere so that these can be addressed constructively. It could also be argued that punitive and negative approaches suggest to staff that they are expected to act irresponsibly. When authority is withheld or removed, the expectation is that one will act in an undesirable manner. Also, the visibility of individual nurses' actions is greatly increased, and may be a source of stress if associated with punitive action. Increased visibility may also make it seem as though there are more mistakes occurring, whereas it may simply be that they are no longer being hidden for fear of punishment. A positive approach is essential: we must recognize that not only are humans fallible, but nursing decisions are usually made on limited information and wrong decisions may be made at times.

'We foster the myth that decision making is based on adequate data collection, but in the real world there is seldom time to do the literature search, thorough family interview, complete physical assessment etc. required for completely adequate data collection. Clinical decision making must consequently admit to the possibility of error' (Manthey 1992).

A plan of care may be unsuccessful for several reasons:

- The patient's condition may be changing rapidly, therefore an associate in conjunction with the charge nurse or another primary nurse may need to change the plan of care.
- Patient outcome may be more dependent on medical care or other extraneous factors.
- There has been a failure to identify problems and goals correctly.

The primary nurse is directly responsible for failures to identify problems and goals, the seriousness of which depends on the level of error and will be different in each case. Primary nurses must be able to demonstrate that they have acted in a way that promotes and safeguards wellbeing and is in the patient's best interests. This must be combined with an appropriate level of competence. The plan will also be judged against what would normally be expected of a primary nurse of a reasonable standard. Tingle (1992c) suggests that this would probably be higher than that expected of an ordinary staff nurse, thereby suggesting that there is increased accountability in primary nursing and also a higher standard of expectation.

Despite further education and development of primary nurses, and support and monitoring of standards by the charge nurse, predicted outcomes may not result and errors may occur. It could be argued that errors are less likely to occur in a system of primary nursing, as:

- the primary nurse has intimate knowledge of the patient;
- the primary nurse receives continuing education and developmental input;
- the primary nurse relies on detailed and documented plans of care;
- responsibility for the total care of a patient is clear;

whereas in a traditional system:

- the charge nurse is most unlikely to have the same level of intimate knowledge about all patients;
- the charge nurse may receive continued education and development but some of the staff nurses may not;
- communication of planned care does not necessarily rely on detailed and documented plans but may be more reliant on oral reporting and ward traditions;
- responsibility for patient care may be fragmented into tasks divided among both trained and untrained nurses, and therefore acts of omission are more likely.

Limitations to responsibility

Even when responsibility is not fragmented, it is difficult to hold a registered nurse accountable for the care a patient receives unless that nurse has commensurate authority and autonomy. It has already been stated that individual nurses are accountable for their own actions. This may be so in terms of specific tasks or aspects of care where they have authority and autonomy. If a nurse was given the responsibility to carry out some aspect of patient care, had the ability to carry it through, but was unable to do so because he/she did not have the authority to see that it happened, it would be difficult to call him/her to account. For example, the charge nurse may have set a ward standard that all patients with a Norton score above 14 should be nursed on a special mattress and have their position changed every 2 hours. The staff nurse is then charged with the responsibility of carrying this out. However, the ward does not have a mattress available and the linen room will not release one without the signature of a charge nurse. Also, the ward is extremely busy and other patients' needs take priority, so that the patient is turned only 3-hourly. The staff nurse does not have the authority to call in an agency nurse, authorize overtime or move staff from another ward. They are, however, obliged to report the situation to their line manager, the senior nurse on duty, who may or may not rectify the shortfall in staffing in order for the standard to be met.

Furthermore, complicated dilemmas may result when the nurse's autonomy is perhaps limited by medical or other staff. A nurse may identify a need for a change from the charge nurse's plan of care, but feel powerless to implement such a change. Their pluralistic accountabilities to themselves, their employer (through the line manger) and the patient are at odds.

Unless nurses have the appropriate balance of responsibility, authority and autonomy they cannot be held accountable for the care of a patient. This is crucial to the success of primary nursing. The balance must be appropriate for all roles at all levels – primary nurse, associate nurse, charge nurse and nurse manager. Different levels of accountability exist within these roles.

Levels of accountability

The associate nurse is accountable to the charge nurse and also to the primary nurse for giving the prescribed care. (Nursing assistants may be responsible for non-nursing duties and, in some cases, for specific aspects of nursing care under the direct supervision of a registered nurse.) The associate nurse must have the authority to change the plan of care should the patient's condition change significantly. (Any changes in care plans are usually made in conjunction with the charge nurse or with another primary nurse, and must be justified to the primary nurse on their return to duty.)

The primary nurse is accountable for the care of a group of patients from admission to discharge, 24 hours a day, 7 days a week. Therefore, primary nurses must have the authority to direct the care of their patients throughout their stay. Primary nurses must have the authority to ensure that care plans are followed when they are off duty – unless there is a change in a patient's circumstances.

The charge nurse is accountable for the quality of care given to a larger group of patients (the ward). The charge nurse must therefore have full authority over management functions within the ward, such as staff recruitment and development, ward staffing (24-hour cover) and the ward budget.

Senior management

Senior nurses in middle management posts usually have authority over a group of wards and for devolving the nursing budget within the unit. However, their autonomy is often undermined if they are not free to make decisions owing to constraints from senior management. Their authority can also be undermined by charge nurses as they seek to increase their authority over their own wards. The responsibility and authority of the middle manager in this system can be unclear, and role definition can be poor (Manthey 1992).

The director of nursing is accountable for the quality of care throughout the institution at all times. The director, then, must have the authority to change to a professional practice delivery system for nursing care. If this authority is denied by other managers, it is difficult to see how the director can be held accountable for the quality of nursing care.

It is also interesting to consider the balance of autonomy, authority and responsibility required and expected for 'named nursing'. A discussion of definitions of named nursing as opposed to primary nursing is beyond the remit of this chapter, but the same considerations for accountability exist. If one accepts that in named nursing patients have the right to know who is in charge of their nursing care, who is responsible and who is accountable, the delivery system and levels of accountability must be addressed. Tingle (1993b) suggests that the named nurse has to be accountable for that patient's care, which requires more than delegated responsibility – rather a nurse with the authority to organize and coordinate care.

CONCLUSION

Accountability in primary nursing is not a muddled 'less talked about the better' issue, but is clearly defined, well articulated and carried through in practice. Siler (1986) proposed that accountability was what distinguished primary nursing from other ways of nursing. Evans (1993) suggests that accountability is of central concern to nurses considering primary nursing.

It may be that primary nursing has embodied the aspirations of nurses as a means of achieving improved quality of care and increasing professionalism. Perhaps they will find other means to achieve the same goals if primary nursing is not available. Primary nursing is not a panacea and will not necessarily be successful in every ward. The commitment and motivation of all nurses involved is essential.

Primary nursing addresses accountability at all levels, and increases the accountability of primary nurses in particular, but also the associate nurse, who is responsible for carrying out a plan of care in the absence of the primary nurse. Associate nurses must also account for their actions, and also for any changes to the plan of care.

It has been argued that primary nursing increases the accountability of nurses to their patients through shared planning, problem solving and an individual approach to care. Increased accountability in primary nursing can only benefit the patient if the increase in nurse autonomy is shared with the patient, and the patient is given a higher-quality service by increasing the visibility of credit and failure and protecting them from poor practice. It will not benefit the patient if increases in nurse autonomy lead to a decrease in patient autonomy; accountability is required without sufficient authority being given; nursing remains highly dependent on an untrained workforce for the delivery of care; nurses are unable to work as primary nurses for organizational reasons (part-time employ-ment or permanent night duty) and become deprofessionalized and deskilled.

The reliance on nursing assistants to deliver a proportion of nursing care needs to be carefully considered. Primary nursing does not require a completely trained workforce, but it undoubtedly functions more effectively with a higher proportion of trained nurses. However, models where nursing assistants are incorporated into the system of primary nursing have been proposed. How much care the primary nurse needs to provide in order to be able to assess, plan and evaluate care effectively is difficult to answer:

'...what amount of care the registered nurse needs to provide in order to remain accountable for overall care is an issue that we in the UK need to address rapidly in the light of the growing numbers of health-care assis-tants' (F. Black 1992).

If a primary nurse provides only 10% of the patient's direct care can he/she be held accountable for the plan of care prescribed? Primary nursing cannot func-tion when the primary nurse is not able to deliver a sufficient proportion of a patient's care, which only he/she can determine as being sufficient. One of the greater hindrances is, perhaps, when only one registered or primary nurse is on duty for the whole ward, with a team of untrained nurses. Although ward situa-tions will vary in needs for skill mix, primary nurses cannot usually fulfil their roles in such circumstances. Again, the total number of patients for whom a primary nurse can reasonably assess, plan and evaluate care will vary according to setting. The success of primary nursing hinges on an individual plan of care negotiated between the primary nurse and the patient. Such individualism, patient empowerment and intimacy is not possible with a large caseload.

The issue of 24-hour, 7-day-a-week accountability has been questioned by Tingle (1992c) as being unrealistic:

'There are legal dangers inherent in the concept of the primary nurse's 24-hour accountability for patient care...Primary nurses can never be totally accountable for the care of their patients' (Tingle 1992c).

Obviously, a primary nurse is not on duty 24 hours a day every day, and nor can he/she personally deliver every aspect of a patient's care. However, it seems anomalous that the accountability of the charge nurse, who also does not work 24 hours every day, has not been questioned on the same premise. The charge nurses set ward policies and procedures using standardized routines to be followed in their absence. A primary nurse sets a plan of individualized care specifically for one patient, to be followed by an associate nurse in his/her absence. It could be argued that primary nursing makes significant steps toward total accountability and avoids many of the problems associated with task and team nursing.

Roles in health care are highly interdependent, therefore absolute account-ability for anything but one aspect of patient care may be an unreasonable goal.

Where a multidisciplinary team shares decision-making in all aspects of care in order to produce an overall care plan, then surely the team becomes accountable for that patient's care? Many teams now have 'key workers' or 'case managers' within the group who coordinate a patient's plan of care and ensure a smooth implementation. Key workers do not usually accept the same level of accountability as primary nurses, owing to the multidisciplinary and coordinating nature of their role. However, case management (Zander 1988) has taken the concept of key worker a stage further by allocating authority and autonomy to the case manager to ensure that planned care in all disciplines is followed. Case managers have usually been nurses, and primary nurses may expand their role to encompass this function, coordinating care throughout the patient's episode of illness regardless of the setting within the hospital.

The named nurse initiative has been briefly considered in relation to primary nursing and accountability. Named nursing must be clearly defined and the accountability associated with primary nursing should not be assumed without mechanisms to ensure appropriate levels of responsibility, ability, autonomy and authority.

If primary nursing achieves nothing else, it certainly encourages nurses to think long and hard about the issue of accountability. A focus on accountability must surely benefit both the public and nursing. However, primary nursing can lead to improvements in patient care which are not simply due to the threat of increased visibility. By decentralizing the hierarchy, nurses gain control of their own actions and become answerable for the consequences. They gain the motivation to achieve things for and with patients, i.e. they become empowered. One must also accept that nurses are fallible. In this system, with increased visibility, names can easily be attached to mistakes as well as to successes. An atmosphere of trust among staff is essential in order to enable them to take anything but the most conservative decisions. If we are not prepared to take some risks, then all that will result is the lowest common denominator of standard care, which must surely be unacceptable to any nurse purporting to be a professional in today's climate.

PART THREE:

Areas of Practice

<table>
<tr><td><h1>Where does the buck stop?
Accountability in midwifery</h1></td><td><h1>6</h1></td></tr>
</table>

Where does the buck stop? Accountability in midwifery | 6

Rosemary Mander

INTRODUCTION

Since the early 1980s nurses have been discussing regularly and authoritatively what accountability comprises. The difficulty in identifying serious midwifery attention being given to this issue is surprising (MIDIRS, 1992). Unfortunately, unlike nurses, midwives do not seem to have shown much serious interest in the subject and accountability has been sadly neglected.

What is the reason for this? Are midwives complacent about their accountability to the extent that it does not merit attention? Although the statement 'Midwives have...the right to be fully accountable' (Roch 1988) may appear to support this, this explanation is unlikely because autonomy, with which accountability is inextricably linked, has been a source of much concern and some research interest to midwives (Mander 1994). Perhaps their anxieties have been focused on autonomy at the expense of accountability? This is a far more likely explanation, particularly in view of midwives' concern about the erosion of their role in the past two decades (Robinson 1990).

This chapter will investigate where midwives currently stand in relation to accountability, drawing mainly on the nursing literature on accountability and comparing it with the situation that has been identified as currently existing in midwifery. Although some may question the relevance of nursing literature to midwives, such material is the most relevant available, and the common nursing background that applies in the UK enhances its relevance.

The discussion of accountability will begin by clarifying the meaning of the term, by briefly focusing on the various meanings that may be applied to it. Next, the vexed question of to whom the midwife is accountable will be addressed. The relationship between the two essential concepts of accountability and autonomy will then be examined. Having provided evidence for the assumption that midwives have yet to become fully accountable for their practice, the chapter will consider what prerequisites are necessary to achieve that state and, finally, look beyond the achievement of full accountability to discuss its implications for midwives.

WHAT IS MEANT BY ACCOUNTABILITY?

This is one of those terms which may be interpreted in a wide variety of ways. Accountability has come to mean almost all things to all people. This may be due to a general uncertainty about its precise meaning, beyond the clearly obvious fact that it has something to do with counting. However, there may be uncertainty about what is being counted and who is doing the counting.

This confusion is discussed by Greenfield (1975) as he attempts to 'gather the diverse strands encompassed by accountability into a more or less coherent form'. The result of his attempt is a focus on organizational accountability and the extent to which US health-care facilities meet the needs of the various interest groups with whom they are associated. Immediately, the distinction between organizational and individual accountability becomes apparent. Unfortunately, no sooner is this distinction clarified than it becomes clouded by contemplation of the huge overlapping areas between the two. This chapter will concentrate mainly on the midwife's individual, or personal, accountability. The implications for the midwife of organizational and institutionalized accountability are inevitably discussed when considering to whom the midwife is accountable, and also the implications of accountability.

Accountability may be defined in terms of 'the formal obligation to disclose what you have done' (Vaughan 1989). Such a definition carries the implication of confessing all on a regular basis. This degree of self-disclosure is quite unrealistic, but considering the potential for disclosure or the preparedness to disclose all would bring us nearer to the meaning of the term.

The concept of preparedness to disclose leads us to Champion's (1991) discussion of accountability in which she emphasizes the sense of being responsible or 'explicable' which it implies. The prerequisite concept of responsibility brings her to discuss the authority for action which it carries, and then on to the need for that action to be within the individual's capabilities and area of expertise. Up to this point, Champion has concentrated on the activity and the circumstances in which it is permitted; the other component of accountability, she identifies, may be found in the need to explain or justify that action. This applies in the sense of making the decision to undertake one course of action as opposed to another, with the implication that the consequences of both are known and understood. The need to explain or justify the choice which was made and the resulting actions may or may not arise, but accountability requires that the individual is always able to provide such explanation or justification. Accountability, therefore, may be seen to be about decision making. The context within which these decisions are made is crucial to being accountable; the individual, working on the basis of their expert knowledge, must be able to exert choice unfettered by trappings or constraints applied by others.

This discussion by Champion is precisely applicable to the role of the midwife in the context of normal childbearing, because it is the midwife who is educated to care for mothers and to anticipate and diagnose deviations from the norm and take appropriate action.

Champion's valuable consideration of accountability is not dissimilar to the meanings drawn by Greenfield (1975). He defines the adjective 'accountable', from which accountability is derived, as: 'subject to giving an account; answerable or capable of being accounted for; explainable'. Like Champion, Greenfield relates accountability and responsibility to the timing of the action. Responsibility is essentially anticipatory: it precedes the action in that it permits the midwife to assume authority for the care that is about to be provided on the basis of expert knowledge and experience. The manner in which that responsibility is manifested is in the accountability of the midwife, which incorporates decision making at the time of the activity and the potential for justifying decisions and actions at some later time.

This distinction in the timing of responsibility and accountability may appear to be little more than academic pedantry, until the implications are considered. Accountability cannot exist without responsibility having previously been granted, accepted and assumed. Whether that responsibility is accepted must depend on the individual midwife in terms of her preparation through education and experience. Thus, a midwife may not be held accountable or have accountability imposed for an action unless she was first given and accepted the responsibility of caring.

In his provocative examination of accountability Etzioni (1975) questions the reality of this phenomenon. He argues to begin with that it may be used symbolically, as little more than a gesture. This serves to establish the moral credentials of the person making the gesture, as for example calling for healthcare providers' greater accountability to their clients. There is, according to Etzioni, no intention of implementing this form of accountability, but it may win over the client/group to the views of the one making the gesture. In a similar vein, Etzioni continues by demonstrating the use of accountability as a ploy in the power politics of health care. He shows that the more powerful an occupational group becomes, the more others are accountable to them. This decidedly cynical approach to accountability may hold more than an element of truth. Its relevance to the context within which midwives work may yet become apparent.

TO WHOM IS THE MIDWIFE ACCOUNTABLE?

Having drawn on the work of Etzioni and Greenfield, which relates more to organizational accountability, it is appropriate to begin this examination of who holds the midwife accountable by considering the institutional and legislative framework within which the midwife works.

Institutional accountability

Although not all midwives in the UK are employed within the NHS or Trusts, a large majority are and some form of institutional accountability is required of them. It is not impossible that even those who work independently may be held accountable to others alongside whom they work. The role of the midwife as an employee inevitably, through a contract of employment, requires adherence to the policies of the organization. Although midwives may perceive their role as being solely to provide care to the woman experiencing normal childbearing, their employers may require an 'extended' expertise in a particular direction, for example in the area of ultrasound investigations (Proud 1988). In the present climate of limited resources, the provision of an ultrasound service by midwives may result in mothers finding that there are fewer midwives available to help, for example, in establishing their breastfeeding. It is necessary to question whether such an example of midwives' accountability to their employers may have adverse implications for the care of mothers and babies.

In historical terms, the major organizational development that had implications for midwives was the introduction of the NHS in 1948 (Robinson 1990). Prior to becoming employed by local authorities and health boards at this time a large majority of midwives had been relatively independent, fully accountable practitioners. The advent of the NHS meant that more women were able and willing to give birth in hospital, and that obstetricians began to become involved in the care of normal, healthy pregnant women. Thus, the orientation of the midwife was changed and midwives' accountability came to be to employers, who now paid a salary, and more and more to obstetrical colleagues. Increasing obstetrical involvement soon led to more monitoring in order to diagnose potential and actual deviations from normal. The need for more hospital facilities, including labour ward beds and postnatal beds, soon became apparent. Perhaps it was in an effort to justify the increasing number of beds in the presence of a falling birth rate that a series of government reports recommended increasing levels of hospital confinement. This scenario escalated and the numbers, status and power of obstetricians increased correspondingly and exponentially. The scene was thus set for the 'technological revolution' which occurred in obstetrics in the early 1970s. This led to the observation that midwives' accountability had been reduced, to the extent that they had been transformed into 'obstetric nurses' (Walker 1972, 1976).

The hierarchical organizations within which midwives continue to work serve only to diminish their accountability, as mentioned by Etzioni (above). It remains, however, to be seen whether the recent publication of the Health Committee Report will provide an opportunity to reverse this trend (Kargar 1992; House of Commons 1992). A twin principle on which this report is founded, together with the mother being the central decision maker, is the need for maternity care to be midwife led. This recommendation clearly carries the potential to increase the midwife's autonomy and accountability.

Accountability to the mother

Legislative accountability was originally intended to protect the public, and the legislative framework within which midwives currently practise continues to have this aim. Although Binnie *et al.* (1984) attempt to distinguish between them, accountability to the public and accountability to the client are synonymous; this is because, logically speaking, the public benefit must include the welfare of the individual mother for whom the midwife is caring. This may not be an easy concept to accept when the overall standard of a mother's care appears to be determined by a book of Midwives Rules and a Supervisor of Midwives.

It may be that accountability to the mother operates in two ways. The mode of operation discussed below, via the legislative framework, may be said to act indirectly by the intervention of human and other agencies. A more direct form of accountability is that which midwives exercise in day-to-day 'hands on' practice involving the care of mothers, babies and families.

Personal accountability

It is cogently argued that in ethical terms the only form of accountability which carries any weight for the midwife is accountability to herself. Tschudin (1989) indicates that this is an unalterable fact of care. Caring, according to one's own philosophy of life, and acting consistently according to the demands set by one's own value system, may call for higher standards than are required by any external agency. Tschudin regards this intensely personal sense of responsibility as comparable with the way 'religious people would say that they have to answer to God'. Supporting this argument, Smith (1981) indicates that this form of accountability operates at all times throughout the life of any health-care provider. It may be that this most personal form of accountability is the highest form, underpinning all others, in that being accountable to oneself is an essential prerequisite to being able to be accountable to anyone else.

While contemplating the significance of personal accountability we should consider the effects of the dichotomy between personal and external accountability on learning. If a care provider makes a mistake, personal accountability would, through reflection, facilitate learning, personal growth and greater maturity. On the other hand, external accountability, through a legislative framework, may lead to little more than disciplinary action.

Legislative accountability

Tschudin (1989), in discussing the various forms that nursing accountability may take, describes the legislative framework through which the nurse's accountability to the public operates. In the opening years of the 20th century the equivalent midwifery framework reached the statute book two decades earlier than nurses', against a background of patriotic public concern at the lack of suitable manpower to fight popular colonial wars. Midwives were considered essential to the provision of a suitably healthy pool of recruits, but the public still needed protection from unsafe and incompetent practitioners. Legislation was sought which would provide adequate protection.

This legislation, which eventually emerged in the form of the first Midwives Act (1902), recognized the special position of midwives compared with other carers, in terms of accountability for their actions. The solitary nature of midwifery practice and the role of midwives in prescribing and administering certain medicines, have been regarded for most of the present century as putting the midwife in need of a specific regulatory framework.

The statutory nature of the Midwives' Rules and the non-statutory but otherwise equivalent code of practice, may cause one to question the extent to which midwives are truly accountable, as these rules relate to clinical care decision-making, among other areas. Newson (1986), having established the original need for the Midwives Rules, as relating to training needs and the protection of families from unsafe practitioners, admits the doubt they cast on midwives' accountability and questions the extent to which they continue to be necessary. In answer, she indicates the variation in midwives' ability, 'from excellent to less than satisfactory'. The existence of 'less than satisfactory' midwives is a sad reflection on our systems of basic and continuing midwifery education and supervision, and is hardly a justification for what may be seen as a legislative straitjacket. Although midwives such as Newson clearly perceive the Rules as a supportive framework within which midwives may practise safely, it may be that the existence of this framework is more of a threat to midwifery by limiting accountability than a support for safe practice.

Closely linked with the Rules and code of practice is the role of the Supervisor of Midwives, described by Isherwood (1988) as monitoring standards and providing advice. The real and potential difficulties in the relationship between the midwife and the supervisor of midwives are described by Isherwood (1989). She maintains that this relationship in a supportive situation may be 'close and cooperative'; it is easy to understand how it may deteriorate into being 'confrontational' when the midwife is called to account to a supervisor for the standard of her practice. She relates how, in such destructive relationships, it is not only the midwife who suffers but also the client, through the poorer service she may be offered.

What has been described as legislative accountability is regarded by some as accountability to the profession (Tschudin, 1989). This certainly does not apply in the context of midwifery, because the legislative framework and associated disciplinary functions are drawn up and operated not solely by midwives but by the UKCC (United Kingdom Central Council for Nurses, Midwives and Health Visitors) (Downe 1989; Flint 1985, 1989, 1990). The question inevitably arises for a traditionally autonomous practitioner such as the midwife, as to whether the existence of these statutory bodies and the associated legislative framework serves to reduce the need for the midwife to regard herself as accountable?

Hierarchy of accountability

It may be argued that personal accountability is the highest order of account-ability. This may be because of the continuing nature of personal accountability or perhaps because of the tendency for the demands we make of ourselves to be higher than those we make of other people. Does accountability on this occasion equate with our conscience? The lower-order forms of accountability, such as the organizational form, may have more easily apparent consequences in terms of the potential for disciplinary action and implications for employment; for this reason they may be more readily discussed and reported. It is suggested here that they pale into insignificance compared to personal accountability.

ACCOUNTABILITY AND AUTONOMY

Some attempt has been made to define accountability and its significance in midwifery (see above). Its relationship with autonomy is close and complex: to disentangle them is no mean feat. It may be that these concepts constitute two sides of the same coin, making them effectively inseparable but still deserving separate scrutiny owing to their differing contributions to informing the midwife's role. Hopefully it will be possible to disentangle the relationship between these concepts in this section.

In the discussion of accountability up to this point it has appeared to be a controlling or limiting phenomenon, to the extent that it may constrain the actions of the practitioner. The possibility of having to explain or justify one's actions carries a strong implication that there is at least the potential for errors to be made. Thus, accountability appears to be a somewhat negative concept. This impression is reinforced by our first glance at the definition of autonomy as 'the power or right of self government' (MacDonald 1981). This definition carries with it the implication that autonomy is a permissive, liberating phenom-enon. It may be regarded as being as positive as accountability is negative; as

Vaughan (1989) observes: 'Some people have interpreted autonomy as meaning total freedom to act'. This clearly cannot apply if chaos is not to ensue.

Some of the limitations to autonomy may be apparent within the dictionary definition. When 'power or right' are conferred or assumed it is necessary to ask 'by whom?' Powers and rights cannot exist in a vacuum, as they carry implications for those who award them as well as others; some negotiation may be necessary before a 'right' is generally agreed.

Vaughan (1989) and Champion (1991) point out other limitations on the 'total freedom' hypothesis. These limitations have been categorized by Hall (1969) according to their internality or externality to the would-be autonomous individual. The former, or 'personal' autonomy, focuses on the way in which autonomy only exists within the boundaries of competence, which are created by the individual's finite knowledge base. The more external form, or 'structural' autonomy, implies the hierarchical or bureaucratic organization within which most midwives practise, and which inevitably limits and constrains their freedom to make decisions.

In an attempt to move forward Hall's established categorization of autonomy, Vaughan (1989) pleads for 'attitudinal autonomy' which relates to individuals' perceptions of themselves as autonomous and accountable practitioners. Attitudinal autonomy may be regarded as having the self-confidence to take appropriate decisions and be prepared to accept the consequences.

A significant contribution to the meagre literature on accountability in midwifery is found in the work of Walker (1972, 1976); the major focus of this research project was the role of the midwife, but it illuminated autonomy in midwife–obstetrician relationships as well as accountability. Walker explores the distinction between the roles of the midwife and the obstetrician. Dictionary definitions succinctly highlight the essential differences: 'midwife' is an Old English term meaning 'with woman', whereas 'obstetrician' originated in the Latin meaning 'to stand before' (MacDonald 1981). This researcher examined their roles by recording semistructured interviews with 49 midwives and 11 medical personnel.

Walker shows how the distinction between roles has become blurred in the minds of some of those involved. This has given rise to conflicts between the expectations and the practice of care. Whereas the midwives saw themselves as responsible for the care of mothers experiencing normal childbirth, the medical staff saw themselves as having overall responsibility and being able to exercise it at will.

Walker invented a hypothetical situation to probe the views of her informants, in which she described an obstetrician walking into a normal birth unrequested; she enquired what the midwife should do and why? Three answers emerged. The first suggested that the midwife should let the obstetrician take over, as care is 'his responsibility'; the second comprised the midwife resentfully letting him take over, taking the view that he should really have left it to her; the third answer involved the midwife continuing with the birth unheedful of his presence.

The first of these answers indicates some carers' limited perception of the accountability of the midwife. This view was supported by the perception that labour is potentially abnormal until safely completed, thus requiring medical supervision at all times. Percival's (1970) infamous dictum that 'Labour is only normal in retrospect' would have provided further support. The midwives, however, considered that they were responsible for care until and unless they sought medical aid. It is apparent that midwives understood the extent to which they were accountable, but that their colleagues were less clear.

It is necessary to question whether the research that Walker undertook in the early 1970s has any continuing relevance? The study by Kitzinger *et al.* (1990) shows that it has, by raising many points which are reminiscent of Walker's much earlier work. Kitzinger *et al.* discuss data which they collected as part of their evaluation of a two-tier system of medical staffing in labour wards. Midwives, senior house officers and consultant obstetricians contributed. Kitzinger argues that the absence of the registrar grade serves to enhance the role of midwives by increasing their decision-making role. The authors comment on the likelihood of obstetricians in a two-tier system having a better understanding of the midwife's ability to practise independently, than the three-tier obstetricians who viewed midwives as 'deputies'.

The work of Robinson *et al.* (1983) involved a wide-ranging examination of the role of the midwife. Questionnaires were distributed to 9200 health-care providers (including midwives, health visitors, GPs and obstetricians) and a sample were interviewed. Data were collected on the views of the various groups concerning the role of the midwife in relation to that of others at the various times in a woman's childbearing career.

Like Walker, Robinson found a considerable grey area when investigating whether a midwife or medical practitioner is the appropriate person to undertake certain aspects of care. The tasks included the booking interview, abdominal examination and making decisions about episiotomy. This work also shows very clearly the extent to which other grades of staff (especially junior medical staff) underestimate the competence of midwives in the areas she examined. These attitudes all too often resulted in the duplication of relatively basic clinical tasks. These recent research projects show that incorrect perceptions of midwives' accountability, first identified two decades ago, still persist.

The autonomy of those involved in the childbearing experience is clearly established in a recent government Health Committee Report, which resulted from the collection of evidence from a vast number and wide range of individuals and organizations from all parts of the UK and from Europe. Although the report (House of Commons 1992) tends to prefer the words 'choice' and 'control', it provides answers to the vexed question of the needs and wishes for autonomy of both mothers and midwives.

This report establishes the autonomy of the mother to the extent that she is to be the central decision maker in matters relating to her care. The other major principle on which this report is founded is the accountability of the midwife, to the extent that all maternity care will be midwife led; the provision for the midwife to consult with obstetricians concerning the relatively small number of mothers in whom problems are identified will continue to feature.

The relationship between autonomy and accountability may be summarized as two concurrent personal monitoring systems. Using the analogy of a continuum of internality/externality, autonomy is more internal while accountability is, perhaps only marginally, more externally orientated. The relationship between autonomy and personal accountability may be so close on this continuum as to be barely perceptible.

PREREQUISITES FOR ACCOUNTABLE MIDWIFERY PRACTICE

The significance of the individual midwife's knowledge base in achieving accountability has already been referred to. Because accountability is about decision making, the knowledge from which those decisions are derived is of fundamental importance. Avoiding the danger of midwives becoming complacent in their knowledge base is similar to the need, emphasized by Champion (1991), for nurses to 'develop and maintain their knowledge'. Midwives, through their long-established system of refresher courses, may have an unfair advantage over nurses in this respect, although it is questionable whether they have made full use of this advantage (Mander, 1986a,b).

The development of the midwifery knowledge base and its nature may also merit attention. For too long this has been founded on personal and occupational experience and medical knowledge (Mander 1992a). The case for a research-based body of midwifery knowledge is put by Houston and Weatherston (1986) on the grounds – they observe regretfully – that 'practice and teaching is [still] based on intuition and experience – not research'. A list of five widely used interventions which 'should be abandoned in the light of the research available' may be used to move this argument forward (Beech 1992). These interventions include time limiting of the second stage of labour, directed maternal pushing, restricting maternal position in the second stage, routine electronic fetal monitoring and offering women soporific medication.

The development of a knowledge base may not in itself be the answer to the problem of becoming fully accountable. The reasons for the non-implementation of research-based knowledge among nurses are manifold and, according to Armitage (1990), may actually derive from accountability being limited by another occupational group.

While traditionally claiming professional status, midwives have tended to ignore the fact that a unique research-based body of knowledge is an essential feature of a profession (Carr-Saunders and Wilson 1933). Bridging the education/theory gap has long been a source of concern to nursing and the other caring professions; similarly, the implementation of research is causing anxiety to researchers and educators. The need for accountability in the presence of an increasingly articulate and autonomous client group should provide midwives with the necessary stimulus to become truly accountable, thereby realizing their claims to professional status.

The close association between nursing and midwifery in the UK carries with it the disadvantage that midwifery has assumed organizational features of nursing which may not be to the benefit of either. An example, demonstrated by Copp (1988), is the hierarchical structure of clinical nursing. Copp maintains that this structure 'indicates a lack of both authority and knowledge' and 'inhibits decision-making at grassroots level'. While nursing attempts to correct this deficiency through the implementation of the nursing process and primary nursing, no such theoretical input to increase individual accountability is being incorporated into midwifery practice. Whether the widespread development of team midwifery (Flint and Poulengeris 1987) may be considered to be a form of 'group accountability' is difficult to assess. The crucial importance of the personal component of accountability, which has been mentioned already, is clearly absent from team midwifery and this deficiency may impede progress towards accountability.

The lack of homogeneity among nurses is identified by Copp (1988) as a factor impeding the development of full accountability. Copp utilizes McClure's (1984) terminology of 'white collar and blue collar nurses' to describe a rift between different levels of nurses, with differing expectations of their work and aspirations to accountability. It is not difficult to imagine how nursing could be shown to be driven in differing directions and how the same argument could equally easily be applied to midwifery. Although individual midwife managers may find it possible to establish a homogeneous working group within a distinct geographical locality, and this approach would establish some degree of group accountability, the problem already discussed in the context of team midwifery remains.

The role of the nurse in care decision making is considered by Copp (1988) to be threatened by their own reluctance to initiate basic aspects of clinical care. She suggests that nurses may be unprepared to take advantage of the accountability they hold for the benefit of their patients. She goes on to warn that certain 'nurse prescribing' opportunities may be assumed by physicians unless they are more effectively utilized. This scenario clearly applies in the midwifery setting where, as has been shown by the work of Robinson et al. (1983), medical practitioners undertake or duplicate the work of midwives.

IMPLICATIONS OF MIDWIFE ACCOUNTABILITY

Although accountability has not been presented as the answer to all of midwifery's problems, this chapter has not yet considered the serious disadvantages which some may prefer not to contemplate. A problem which would arise, were midwives to assume full accountability, is that their employers would cease to accept vicarious liability as at present through the employer–employee relationship. Midwives being fully accountable would mean their being answerable to their clients for the decisions taken prior to providing care. The spectre of litigation assumes a more solid form and more awe-inspiring dimensions when a one considers that midwives, like their medical colleagues, may be held personally responsible for any perceived or actual errors of care. Without a willingness to accept this ultimate responsibility, it is not possible for midwives to regard themselves as fully accountable. Having raised the spectre of litigation, midwives' responsibilities in improving the present complaints system become apparent. Were this system less confrontational, as suggested in the Health Committee Report, this grotesque phenomenon of litigation would assume more manageable proportions.

Like Copp, Vaughan (1989) emphasizes that there may be a price to pay for accountability, i.e. the cost of taking risks, personally, professionally and organizationally, and accepting the consequences of our own actions. Risk taking is an essential component of learning and the personal growth that ensues; for this reason accountability is as essential for the maturation of midwifery into a genuine profession as it is for each individual midwife to become genuinely professional.

CONCLUSION

Drawing largely on the nursing literature, this chapter has considered the position of midwives in relation to accountability. The multiplicity of agencies to whom midwives may be held accountable suggests that their accountability is severely curtailed by the legislative framework within which they practise. Research focused more on midwives' declining autonomy has shown that their accountability is similarly threatened. Midwives, through their organization of education and research, have it within their power to correct this serious deficit in their professional role, but before seeking to assume complete accountability midwives must be comfortable with the increased personal responsibility this would require them to bear.

In summary, it is clear that midwives are moving forward in the direction of greater accountability. In this journey they have both help and hindrances, some of which require action by midwives themselves.

Accounts, accounting and accountability in psychiatric nursing

7

Stephen Tilley

INTRODUCTION

This chapter relates the topic of accountability in psychiatric nursing to face-to-face interaction with patients and colleagues. It begins with a brief discussion of the centrality of the topic and an introduction of the concepts 'account', 'accounting', and 'accountability' as working words. These concepts are then explored with reference to both the literature and the author's research.

The centrality of the topic

The topic of accountability is central to psychiatric nursing in four ways. First, accountability is an aspect of the shared life which nurses and patients confront daily by virtue of participation in a society which increasingly stresses members' rights and obligations – as providers and consumers of health care and other goods and services; as participants in civic, school, local authority or national decision-making. In various institutions, people encounter systems and mechanisms designed to devolve responsibility for decision-making to an organizational level and, ultimately, to someone who can be asked to account for what has been done or not done in terms of finance, decision-making or professional judgement. Psychiatric nurses and those they help alike face these common demands for accountability.

Secondly, psychiatric nurses, being employed in institutions, are accountable to their managers. They are obliged to produce for a third person a 'trace' of their interaction with a second person with whom they are engaged in some form of social action. The UKCC (1989) advised that 'a registered practitioner: is accountable for her actions as a professional at all times'; and that 'in situations where the practitioner is employed she will be accountable to the employer for providing a service which she is employed to provide and for the proper use of the resources made available by the employer for this purpose'. Managers, like the bureaucrats described by Raffel (1979), cannot be present at the action, and rely on accounts to know what has been done.

Thirdly, accountability is central to psychiatric nursing. Nurses registered with the UKCC practise in light of the Council's guidelines on exercising accountability: 'practitioners...ensure that the reality of their clinical environment and practice is made known to and understood by appropriate persons or authorities, doing so as an expression of their personal professional accountability exercised in the public interest' (UKCC 1989).

The Council notes: 'The words 'accountable' and 'accountability' each occur only once in the code, both being found in the stem paragraph out of which the subsequent 14 clauses grow. They do, however, provide its central focus...'. The Council notes the need 'to establish more clearly the extent of accountability of registered nurses' 'to assist them in the exercise of professional accountability'. Accountability is thus not a fixed attribute but rather something realized in practice: 'an integral part of professional practice' related to 'mak(ing) judgements in a wide variety of circumstances and (being) answerable for those judgements'.

The UKCC can go only so far in clarifying for what, to whom and under what circumstances the nurse as professional is accountable. The Council 'does not seek to state all the variety of circumstances in which accountability has to be exercised' but instead states 'important principles', e.g. 'the primacy of the interests of the public and patient or client...'.

Fourthly, psychiatric nurses may be accountable to researchers or professionalizers. Researchers into psychiatric nursing in Britain have repeatedly concluded that nurses are not able to tell what they do in a way that makes their practice visible and recognizable as accountable professional practice.

Altschul (1972) reviewed American texts claiming that a patient–nurse relationship is (prescriptively) founded on interaction characterized by the nurse's deliberate, purposeful action and use of words. She asked British nurses to tell about their interaction with patients, and concluded that they were not practising on the basis of an 'identifiable perspective'. In terms of the UKCC's guidelines such nurses could be seen as not being answerable for their judgements, not providing explanations that made sense (to the researcher).

The nurses claimed that their actions were 'common sense', but that sense was not apparent to Altschul. In the variety of circumstances in which they worked, the basis of their action was not evident. Cormack (1976) found psychiatric nurses similarly unable to account for their interaction with patients. More recently, Wooff and Goldberg (1988) criticized community psychiatric nurses' case management practices, implying that resources for health care must be accounted for.

Thus, researchers and policy makers question nurses' ability to account effectively for their practice, in contexts defined by the researchers and policy makers themselves. Given the centrality of the topic, it is important to have a working understanding of the terms 'account', 'accounting' and 'accountability' that is useful to psychiatric nurses.

In the following sections, these concepts are related to themes of knowledge, power and moral order in psychiatric nursing (*cf.* Tilley (1995) on which the argument of this chapter is based). An argument is developed in three parts:

- When giving and receiving accounts, nurses and patients draw on, reproduce and negotiate frames of meaning.
- Processes of accounting structure and are structured by 'working relationships' – accounting construed as practices of explanation and attribution of responsibility for action.
- Accountability entails an obligation to participate in processes of accounting and hence the production and reproduction of moral orders.

ACCOUNTS

A shift in meaning

It is essential to understand nurses' accounts, accounting and accountability from an empirically grounded perspective, yet there has been little empirical research on psychiatric nurses' accounting practices. Researchers have typically taken nurses' accounts for granted as unproblematic windows on practice (Cormack 1976; MacIlwaine 1980, 1983). Here it will be argued that accounts can better be regarded as forms of social practice which reflexively constitute the nurses' work.

Altschul's (1972) use of the term 'account' in a highly influential research-based text offers a useful point of departure for exploring the concept:

'If nurses were asked to account for their interactions, junior nurses by senior nurses, and all nurses by doctors, if senior nurses were encouraged to make explicit what at present is being done without insight, a great deal of existing skill would become observable, and some lack of skill would be remedied. There seems to be an urgent need for a deliberate and conscious effort to increase communications and to increase observability of patients by nurses, of nurses by each other, and between nurses and doctors. Only then can the necessary theoretical background for effective interaction with patients become available.'

Envisaged here were a system of accounting and a structure of accountability which would somehow make the work of nurses observable to those above, and thereby subject to social control. Accounts are reified as aspects of a hierarchical system which could, in some fairly straightforward way, deliver the goods in understanding psychiatric nursing. A limitation of this understanding of accounts is that it ignores the problem of interpretation of what is being done, and the related problems of understanding local culture and frames of meaning.

An alternative, interpretative understanding can be found in Harré's (1979) notion of accounts as devices for 'smoothing rough passages in social life':

> 'If rough passages in social action are smoothed over by accounting, then lack of skill in accounting is sure to lead to a troubled life for the individual with that deficit. Perhaps one of psychiatry's functions is to provide more powerful accounting material as well as a measure of improved skill in using it. It may be that psychiatry could be a more potent technique if its practitioners made more deliberate efforts to amplify both resources for and skill at accounting.'

Construed thus, accounts could play a role in psychiatric nursing different from that imagined by Altschul. Patients would be regarded as people unable to account for what they do, encountering 'rough passages' and dependent on others, including nurses, to provide accounts or 'smooth the passages'.

From such an interpretive perspective (Denzin 1989; Schutz and Luckmann 1974; Harré, 1979), accounts are regarded as discursive events which interpret the situation and order action within it. They are called for and given when some question arises about the ongoing social action, threatening to disrupt it, and are given primarily so that practical action can proceed. Accounts make features of settings 'seeable and reportable, i.e. accountable' for practical purposes (Garfinkel 1968). Thus Lyman and Scott (1970):

> 'By an account...we refer to a statement made by a social actor to explain unanticipated or untoward behaviour – whether that behaviour is his own or that of others, and whether the proximate cause for the statement arises from the actor himself or someone else.'

Patients can be regarded (Tilley 1995) as persons who interact with nurses because they cannot account for their experience or behaviour. They have 'strayed' from the paramount reality of everyday life and the common-sense world (*cf.* Berger and Luckmann 1967). Nurses' work is regarded, from an interpretative and discursive perspective, as action motivated to answer (give accounts in response to) the questions 'Why is this patient here?' and 'What do we have to do for him or her?'.

Accounts, theories and frames of meaning

Revision of the concept of 'account' for psychiatric nursing entails readdressing the problem of common sense.

Accounts given and received in practice settings are 'warrantable understandings from within a frame of reference' (Shotter 1984), related primarily to the frame of common sense rather than theory. That the frame of reference in practice is, typically, not a theoretical frame needs to be emphasized, given the current push to make psychiatric nursing a theory-driven discipline (Reynolds and Cormack 1990). Accounts are primarily practical devices which name things as what they are, not in theoretical terms (Shotter 1984).[1]

Practically, nursing is fundamentally concerned with the activities of daily living, the myriad everyday things that people might do in relation to health, illness or dying had they the necessary 'strength, will and knowledge' (Henderson 1978). The ordinary, lay and everyday have been denigrated or rendered invisible in previous research on psychiatric nursing, which has emphasized the non-ordinary, professional and theoretical dimensions of nursing practice. This may be due largely to the role of nursing research in promoting professionalization (Tilley, in press). Neglect of common sense has to be redressed if psychiatric nurses' accounts are to be understood as legitimate accounts of their work.

Competence and accounts in psychiatric settings

The issue of competence in psychiatric nursing is two-edged. One aspect concerns patients' competence to account for their actions, and the other nurses' competence to account for their practice.

Shotter (1984) argues that social competence depends on the ability to account for how one makes one's actions 'conformable to common sense' rather than theory. Competence in accounting is itself a form of social competence, which may be limited if a person's stock of social knowledge is inadequate (for example if the patient has, through illness or institutionalization, lost contact with ordinary life, its activities and the ways of accounting for it).

Goffman (1967) construed psychiatric symptoms as violations of social order, which generally call for some kind of account (*cf.* Lyman and Scott 1970). The frame of reference that psychiatric patients draw on to make sense is often not shared by nurses: it does not conform to common sense (*cf.* Beck 1976). For example, the author (Tilley 1995) was told by a student nurse who had accompanied a patient during a panic attack: 'what's everyday for us is not for her', i.e. the everyday frame of reference was not shared by the patient and the nurse.

The second aspect of competence relates to psychiatric nurses' accountability for action. If the 'real' basis for psychiatric nursing accountability is not established, nurses risk being seen as incompetent or non-competent. Empirically (Tilley 1995), nurses' competence in accounting was based on their ability to identify what was responsible for a patient's behaviour – an illness, or the patient being a willing agent. Thus a nurse gave an account of a meeting with a patient and his wife:

'**Nurse:**...In previous Kardexes it had been said there was something underlying between the wife, and, (the patient), right? Em, so I just thought, Well, I'll see if there's anything I can pick up, (?), eh, seeing if they have any, (?), (?) having problems. Em... (They) both denied that there was any real problems, just the basic, sort of everyday, husband and wife, problems, right? Eh, and then it came out that, the main problem was, em, (the patient's) relationship with his son....That was the major problem at the time. (?Right.) It didn't actually relate to his illness, or why he was here, but it was a ma-, well, in a way it did, because he was worried about it, right? Uh, it was one of his major worries.'

Interpretation (and in some cases negotiation and determination) of responsibility is a main part of the work in interaction between psychiatric nurses and neurotic patients. Accounts are the devices through which the work on responsibility is reflexively accomplished. In the following excerpt, the definition of what was responsible for a patient being in the admission ward was discussed by a nurse:

'**Nurse:** So, as such, we weren't really, being pushed to, offer her, treatment for, the panic attacks. She's had some generalized literature, uh, the psychologist had a chat with her, but apparently her problem was alcohol, not, anxiety...'

The patient's responsibility for work on (to tackle or look at) the problem was determined in interaction:

'**Nurse:** (? In a), nature of, the way she seems to look at things she doesn't seem to be really challenging much, you know, letting lots of things go past, without really looking at them and saying an opinion on things. And she's obviously, not wanting to, too deeply, really at anything, even her cure, you know, if you could call it that, of being here, (?) we're, we're saying 'This will work', but, she seems to be willing just to take that pretty much at face value. Which I, I feel is, indicates that, indicates that she herself's not really going to be able to cope, and that these issues, that she's not tackling, will probably cause anxiety, which will cause other issues, to be not (sniggers) tackled... 'E-, everything's fine at home, it's just these, symptoms that is the problem.'...Uh if, if you, put a question, over, and in the question you'd, in-built, you know, an opener, let u-, say (? you), 'Do you not feel that it could be, situation at home that might be...adding to, your anxiety?' If you get a straight 'No' from that, then obviously you can not move any further. Whereas, if, 'Well, there are some things that are problems', and (chuckles) then you say 'Well, what kind of problems?', then you can move in from there, but, as long as 'Everything, at home is fine, there is nothing wrong', then obviously, she's not willing to look at that...(?We) may get rid of her symptoms, the things at home may continue on, but, she might not develop any psychiatric type symptoms, she might just (laughs) end up with a broken marriage, which, a lot of people, encounter without actually engaging in, contact with the psychiatric services.'

This excerpt illustrates that accounts not only entail, but are, interpretations of social action. Accounts are forms of social action that accomplish attribution of or relief from responsibility for social action. Thus they realize – i.e. make real and enable others to grasp – social acts. Accounts may be given and heard as claims about what or who is responsible for some situation; as such they may be refuted. These characteristics generally have particular force in the negotiation of social reality in psychiatric settings, and specifically in determinations of whether a patient is ill or 'really ill', or has problems, these being the working definitions of psychosis and neurosis in psychiatric settings (see below).

Accounts, common sense and professional judgement

Accounts, considered as devices for attributing responsibility (Lyman and Scott 1970) and for conveying the rationality of commonplace activities (Garfinkel 1967; Hughes 1980; Baruch 1981), are important in formal processes of decision-making, judgement and labelling. The function of patients' and nurses' stories in nursing assessment and practice is similar to that in jury trials (Bennett and Feldman 1981). Accounts in the form of stories are often used by patients and nurses to convey those features of situations which must be grasped if social judgements about agency and responsibility are to be made.

Judgements of responsibility hinge on attributions of motive conveyed through accounts and stories. The common-sense concept of deviance (McHugh 1968) entails a judgement that the person accused of a deviant act knew what he/she was doing and could have done otherwise. Accounts are implicated in judgements of deviance[2] and illness (Smith 1978).

Diagnosis itself can be regarded as a form of accounting. The premise here is that, if a person fails to play his or her role as an agent, an account is required to be given by that person or another. Conventionally, professionals have the exclusive right to give certain kinds of accounts (e.g. only doctors may give accounts of illness based on diagnosis). Hence, from this perspective professionals play a part in the maintenance and repair of social order and in the practices of social control (Parsons 1951; Turner 1987).

Practically, then, the 'recognition' of illness entails legitimation. In the sites studied by Tilley (1995), patients who would be accounted for in a diagnostic framework (e.g. the International Classification of Diseases) as neurotic were regarded as 'not ill' or 'not really ill', but rather as having problems (*cf.* Towell 1975). Psychotic patients were regarded as ill. The common-sense meaning was that the patient who was ill or really ill was not responsible for his or her behaviour, whereas the patient with problems was responsible for working on them. If patients declined to work on their problems, the point of dispute became whether they could not or would not do so. In short, the issue became whether that person was really an agent, able but unwilling to work, or a patient, unable to do so. Their legitimacy as a patient was thus negotiated by means of the accounts given by and about them. An implication of this is that patients who were ill could not be expected to provide an account of their actions, whereas those with problems could.

Taxonomy of psychiatric patients' and nurses' accounts

Lyman and Scott (1970) provide a taxonomy of accounts. These include excuses – which acknowledge that something wrong has been done, but that one is not to be considered responsible; and justifications, given when wrongdoing is denied. This taxonomy is relevant to understanding empirical data on psychiatric patients' and nurses' accounts (Tilley 1995).

Patients provided accounts in which they distinguished between social talk, that is, talk about what they shared with nurses, which was unremarkable: topics such as clothing, make-up, holidays, women's things; and 'illness talk' or 'problem talk', that is, talk about what was not shared, what had brought them to the admission wards.

The patients spoke as if they had to provide an account of why they were there, to participate in a system of accounting which constituted the work of the admission wards - providing diagnoses construed as excuses from responsibility (*cf.* Parsons 1951). Patients were sometimes not able to excuse their inability to carry out their everyday roles, and sometimes depended on nurses and other professionals to provide them with an account, which could be withheld. Nurses' and patients' accounts of the same phenomenon in some cases differed (Tilley 1995). The main narrative line was often the same, but the patient's action was interpreted differently by patient and nurses.

Patients commonly gave accounts of 'not wanting to' and 'inability to bring oneself to', both to nurses in interaction and in telling a researcher about their conversations with nurses. Thus a patient explained to the author (Tilley 1995):

> '**Researcher:** Um, (Note: researcher is reading text of first account) w-w-, yeah, when you were ill, here, you felt dizzy on your feet, and you couldn't do much, you didn't feel like doing much.
> **Patient:** Well I didn't want, well,
> **Researcher:** Right.
> **Patient:** Couldn't.'

Disputes between nurses and patients often focused on 'can't do or won't do?'. Thus a student nurse gave the following account of a patient:

> '**Nurse:** (My) reaction to that (Note: to what the patient said) was (the patient) was maybe wanting to go home and bring a sorta suitcase in and,

reinforce her ideas that she wanted to stay a while...Um, without saying 'assumption', I had it mind that because of, em, her, sort of, her unwillingness to stay away from the hospital while she was, actually a patient at a different hospital...she still kept coming back here. And at every given opportunity gave reasons why she should still be in hospital, as inpatient. That's why I presumed that, you know, this was another ploy of, of needing to stay in.'

Accounts may also provide occasions and devices for negotiating responsibility:

'**Nurse:**...she (the patient)...told me how her weekend had gone and she felt that the drugs had a lot to do with it and (I) let her know that the drugs really didn't have much to do with how she had been at home, eh, it was mainly up to her, a lot of it was up to her. And she says well, you know, 'Do you think that's, you know, do you not think it is the drugs?', I said 'No, I think I think a lot's something to do with you and you've got to try maybe to get on with Phil (Note: husband)...'

Nurses, when asked to account for their interactions with patients, likewise offer excuses and justifications. The following is a nurse's justification of taking a 'tough line' towards a patient:

'**Nurse:** We decided that, we'd, stop being as supportive, eh, changed our attitude in a way that, although we were still being supportive, we're really, weaning her off us, if you see what I mean, so, like she was saying 'I cannae cope with any more passes' and I was saying 'Well you're going on pass, (? like more) sort of thing' (laughs). Sort of more, strict (?) the tough, yeah, more the sort of tough line you sometimes have to take if, they're too dependent. It, it's (? a line or ? one) we, occasionally take, with over-dependent patients, eh, so that they'll go back into the community.'

The justification established by the (tacit) assumption that return to the community was a good thing could excuse what might have sounded uncaring.

The following account (Tilley 1995) of a nurse's inability to interact as she would have liked constitutes an excuse:

'**Nurse:** I felt that, (?) during the Kardex I was running after Mary most of the time, and Elsa was lying on the floor, but P4 was there too, you know, she was there, but like I didn't have any time at all with her, and she was sitting crying, so I said that, basically to let her know that I, I was still speaking to her...And, eh, let her know that I was, I was noticing her.'

In this excerpt, reference to circumstances provides the basis for excuse.

It is important to recognize that informal accounts of justification and excuse given in, and necessary for, the smooth running of practice may not accord with the principles that guide the production of formal accounts of nurses' work

(Kardex entries, reports and input to planning meetings). Nurses in practice have to take account of informal frames of reference in the moral orders of everyday ward work. Thus, a charge nurse in one site said that the management priorities were to ensure that patients were 'safe, fed, and happy, in that order' (Tilley 1995). To be considered acceptable, accounts had to fit with these priorities. Thus, it would have been inappropriate for a nurse to have attempted to justify having been engaged in a one-to-one therapeutic talk with a patient while another patient was absconding.

Accounts, ordinary judgement and professional judgement

Accounts may bridge ordinary judgement and professional judgement by conveying the ordinary judgement necessary for professional judgement (Hughes 1980). The concept of 'excuse from responsibility', already discussed, mediates commonsense judgements and medical and nursing judgements of illness (Hughes 1980, 1988; Turner 1987).[3]

Tilley (1995) suggests that psychiatric nurses are involved in the social processes of accounting through which patients either are or are not excused from responsibility. Nurses make judgements about whether patients' accounts accord with common sense, thereby establishing whether the complaint is evidence of a problem or indicative of illness. One of the problems psychiatric patients often face is their inability to give accounts of their actions, experience and planning which accord with common sense (Beck 1976) or common discourse principles (Bennett and Feldman 1981; Harré 1983). Similarly, they become the subjects of accounts given by others which show their deviation from the norms of common sense (Smith 1978).

On the basis of their 'readings' of patients' accounts, nurses exercise discretion in providing care (*cf.* Adler and Asquith 1981). Their accounts of what they are doing may be read as displaying the nurses' competence in the practical settings.

Thus, as devices for determining responsibility, through explanation, justification and excuse (Lyman and Scott 1970), nurses' and patients' accounts provide both the occasions for and the means of moral reasoning. This reasoning may entail showing the accordance of action with practice ideologies.[4]

Accounts and working ideologies

In acting accountably both nurses and patients referred to what may be regarded as 'working ideologies' about responsibility for problems (Tilley 1995). They did so in accounts of what was responsible for the appearance of the patient at the time ('Why is she here now?') which articulated with accounts of the staff's responsibilities toward the patient. Such accounts contained an analysis of the patient's powers and liabilities and the staff's powers. For example, an experienced nurse in one site talked about a patient's problem:

'**Nurse:** ...So we tried to talk with her, to try and find out what this was. And, between ourselves and the medical staff came up with this idea, that uh, probably it was something fairly long-standing...and, there was a lot of anxiety that she had which was put off, on these panic attacks so, so (? it was) thought, to bring in the psychologist to try and handle it from there, and, basically we then saw it as being simply a management of building up her confidence, and having nurses available to work with her, on her programme.'

Working ideologies were drawn on to legitimate the allocation of professional and interpersonal responsibility – or (*cf.* Peplau 1978), the allocation of the patient's responsibility for work and the staff's responsibility for work with the patient. The work and the working relationships thus constituted, were related reflexively to definition of an indexical 'it'[5] and work on 'it'. In one site, for example, the nurses constructed themselves and the patients in terms of 'availability for work'. The patient was required to be available for work on 'it', that is, on her problems. Availability of the resources of the site – expressed in terms of time – was dependent on the patient's availability for work. The nurses' strategies of work management and accounting practices, and their accountability, were based on this notion of availability for work on 'it'. Such a working ideology, in this case one of responsibility, can be read for its implicit or explicit theory of the patient as a person (agent or patient) as well as for what it implies about the appropriate working relationship between patient and nurse (*cf.* Towell 1975). The ideology was drawn on to structure face-to-face interaction and to order work, to set priorities and to tell self and others what was to be done.

Paradigm and template accounts

There has been very little work on the typical form and content of psychiatric nurses' accounts considered as situated social practices.

Accounts may vary from site to site. In one site Tilley (1995) found that the typical or template accounts were based on 'being available' for patients, or on 'giving patients opportunities'. These implied a high degree of patient responsibility for obtaining or refusing help. In another site the nurses appeared, in their own and patients' accounts, as 'middlemen'. Their role was to support the definition of the work of others and others' definitions of 'it'. Participation in the giving of such accounts entailed risks: the nurses at the second site did not command the definition of the patient as 'work object' (Stacey 1976), and were liable to be relegated to a service role.[6]

Nurses may draw on varied and sometimes contradictory accounting forms and styles to interpret and justify their practice. Nurses working within a system of accountability based on a working ideology of availability could represent themselves as potentially but not actually responsible, by representing the patient as responsible. Hence the following account of mutual non-legitimation (*cf.* May and Kelly 1982; Tilley 1995):

> '**Nurse:** (Our role has been) initially assessing. And then, as I say, reassurance and generally trying to engage with her, to give her the opportunity to talk over these issues, which have been raised, but which she is not wanting to do any work on. Um, involvement also with the support group, again, to give her opportunity to vent her feelings and think through the issues, which again have not really been taken up. Um, latterly, as I say, we've withdrawn a bit to a more broadly supportive role....She's signalled to us she's not really wanting to engage in anything terribly deep in the way of conversation, so, time for exploratory work you could say's now no longer available, so (?that) it's just building her up emotionally.'

Different nurses working in the same site could draw on different ideologies to form alternative views. For example, another nurse gave the following account about the same patient:

> '**Nurse:** In the support group...there were things, I don't think she said, in the family situation, that she didn't always express her feelings outside in the, family, and that was one thing we talked about in the group....In the support group...she also found that she could talk, through the support group she learned that she could, talk to other patients as well, you know, other people...saying that, uh, that it was sorta good to be able to talk to other people and share experiences here...'

Different nurses conveyed a different sense of their power in face-to-face interactions, drawing on different frames of meaning (e.g. 'responsibility' versus 'sharing') to explain interaction. They drew on different ideologies in accounting for the interaction.[7] The frames of meaning reflected both common experiences, for example the experience of sharing, and ideologies shared by nurses in the site. Nurses drew on specialist or technical frames of meaning (related, for example, to illness) to structure and account for specific interaction (such as a 'programme' for agoraphobia). The view of the patient as a person likewise differed in different accounts of the working relationship based on different frames of meaning or ideologies.

Some psychiatric nursing texts are now providing more formal template accounts, giving what might be seen as typical or ideal forms and contents for nurses' accounts of their practice. The template accounts provided by Ritter (1989) in a psychiatric nursing procedures manual include a research-based rationale for psychiatric nursing actions, followed by step-by-step descriptions of the action involved and practice-based rationales for the actions. These are templates for accounts of psychiatric nursing as reasoned, deliberate action.

With regard to the form of accounts, Tilley (1995; in press) found that the typical account was a story of 'work', with six elements: the patient; the point in the patient's stay (the episode of admission or care); the site at the time; the problem or illness; the remedy; and the narrating nurse's voice.

ACCOUNTING

Accounts are to accounting as given conversations are to the wider conversation that structures social and personal being (*cf.* Harré and Gillett, 1994). Accounts have been discussed in terms of the production of knowledge and social reality. Accounting may be seen as a process – the Kardex, the student nurse's process recording, ward rounds, handovers, the night report, talk to friends, self or the 'generalized other' – that operates through individuals, thereby constituting them.

Accounts are structured in systems and processes of accounting. If accounts in psychiatric nursing are answers to the questions 'Why is she here now?' and 'What do we have to do for her?', the commonsense version of accounting is the process of nurses and patients asking and answering the questions over time. If accounts are devices for realizing what the main thing to do with a patient is, that is, as modes of knowledge, then accounting should be interpreted in terms of power – who structures the processes of accounting; who can require that accounting be done?

Accounting is a form of labour (not usually costed, except informally – for example, the consultant in one site was anxious that nurses' record keeping would take too much time) and can change the value of labour, in the sense that constitution of a more highly valued social act can be accomplished through re-accounting for the same behaviour. Thus, in second-order accounts nurses sometimes shifted from saying that they had 'noticed' something, to saying 'my observation was...', the use of the term 'observation' indicating deliberate nursing action which enhanced the value of what they had done.

Each system of accounting is a solution to the problem that there is something to be accounted for and that somebody has an interest in that something. The something might be numbers of patients in the ward (in case of fire); the current state of symptoms; or 'the problem', 'it', the answer to the question 'Why is she here now?'. Systems of accounting are indeed predicated on there being something to be accounted for: nurses and patients enter into interaction in an admission ward with the assumption that there is a reason for the patient being there, and the problem is to find out what that reason is.

Formal and informal accounting

As there are formal and informal accounts, so there are formal and informal systems of accounting. Formal systems, in which accounts are structured to provide a systematic means of inscription and recovery of knowledge about the patient, are increasingly evident. These may include systems of audit, standard setting and monitoring, care planning and review. Whatever the formal systems, there will undoubtedly also be informal ones which the practitioners know they need to maintain if their work is to proceed. As Garfinkel (1967) noted, everything in an organization is 'none of somebody-else-in-that-organization's business'.

Examples of formal systems of accounting include the Kardex, handover, one-to-one therapy and group therapy, case conferences and ward rounds. Each system of accounting opens up some individual or group to some other individual or group for some form of interrogation (Carl May, personal communication), even if that is as benign as 'How are you?' (see, in the previous section, the quotation in which the nurse described 'trying to engage with (the patient), to give her the opportunity to talk...' , and the patient 'not really wanting to engage in anything terribly deep in the way of conversation, so time for exploratory work you could say's no longer available...'). The patient was implicitly criticized for not taking part in the system of accounting in which the nurses attempted to enrol her. This example indicates that accounting is a system of discipline (*cf.* Foucault 1982). Each such system can spawn forms of resistance to surveillance.[8]

Resistance

Systems of accounting are systems of power. Power, conceived as the production of various effects, including truth effects, and operating at the 'capillaries' of systems of domination (Foucault 1982), becomes evident when resisted.

In general, formal systems of accounting in psychiatric nursing 'manage out' the nurse's interpretative work. The desired documents are 'objective' and objectifying. Likewise, systems of accounting in psychiatric nursing typically manage out the 'emotional labour' (Hochschild 1983) which nurses do to sustain relationships and the organization. Formal systems of accounting can be seen in the case noted above, where the charge nurse noted the process of deciding, through processes of referral and assessment, whether drink or anxiety was the problem.

Informal accounting has been found to be tied up with issues of control, power and legitimation (Tilley 1995). Power in interaction could be 'read' from accounts involving responsibility-construction which centred on judgements of 'can't do or won't do?' and 'needs help or wants help?'. Thus a patient claimed that she 'needed' the nurses to 'trigger' her because she could not think for herself and blamed this on her illness. Her account was countered in a nurse's account:

> '**Nurse:** ...when Patient 2 was first in and was actually quite ill, she wouldn't lead a conversation, and she required a lot of prompting which, now, and from that conversation in particular she certainly didn't need.'

The patient's claim that her untidiness had to be excused was not accepted by the nurse:

> '**Nurse:** ...she seemed quite willing to lead conversation and very quickly (? for) around to 'I'm fed up being in these clothes' and I said 'I sympathize with that, because (?they of ?we) don't like to be in the same clothes all the time but at least, you don't need to have dirty clothes' and reminded her of the washing facilities.'

A series of excerpts shows another patient involved in systems of accounts which made her subject to social control of her everyday activities and the enforcement of the 'paramount reality of everyday life' (Berger and Luckmann 1967; *cf.* Chapman 1987 and Bloor and Fonkert 1982). Ordering of her time and activity was legitimated as 'work', 'therapy', the 'programme'.

The patient, complaining that she was anxious at not having enough time to get to a wedding, had asked the nurses' permission to leave the ward early. The nurses refused, saying that she was obliged to attend a ward meeting. The patient complained that staying back to attend the meeting would increase her anxiety. The nurses refused to accept that the delay involved could account for her anxiety. A trained nurse drew on her knowledge of the actual time it would take to get to the wedding, and said:

> '**Nurse:** I told my colleagues, and...they were of the impression too, that, there was more to it than just the fact, that she wasn't getting, away early...she was, overly upset over, such a, seemingly (sniggers) trivial fact....'

Another nurse gave the following account of the same incident:

> '**Nurse:** What we were trying to do? Trying to get her to, to recognize, the fact her, her worries (?), that, there's, there is nothing wrong to be, in being worried, or apprehensive, about what she was, (? about to face), although it was a happy occasion, being a wedding, uh, but e-, even I think for most people, large gatherings, weddings, parties, it can sometimes be, quite nerve wracking, for a lot of people, it can, and there's nothing, wrong with a-, admitting it. Trying to focus in, on, what it was.'

A third account of the episode from another experienced member of the nursing staff:

> '**Nurse:** We had persuaded Patient 4 to attend the support group and then go through to, to uh, Glasgow, after the support group, which still gave her plenty of time....And, when we got to the support group, in fact, Patient 4 still had some anxiety, 'churning in her stomach' as she called it, but, was saying how, she would in fact at that point in, on the Friday afternoon, might have been quite happy if somebody had told her not to go at all. So I think this sort of indicating her, ambivalence or her, her desire to be told what to do....'

While interpretations and warrants were required at every point in the interaction and in accounting for it afterwards, nurses and patients had different rights and obligations in systems of accounting. The nurses could oblige the patient to stay; their apology was discretionary.

The power involved in accountable interaction is also reflected in accounts in which patients judged, excused and justified the nurses. Thus the patient who was the subject of the accounts just cited later said of herself:

> '**Patient:** (One of the nurses) actually thanked me for staying on, which said a lot for her, and, I was quite honest as well, I said that, well I had stayed on but I did admit that I was, very upset and I was quite angry at Phyl, so I told her that...So I, I feel the air was cleared a bit and, I'm glad I did get on OK and, everything's back to normal again. With the staff, not that they were, they possibly were angry with me as well, and thought I was being, acting a bit young for my age, but, it's just it was pure emotion and excitement.'

The same patient gave the following account of herself and another patient:

> '**Patient:** I just feel a great load's been lifted off me and I can see now, probably a lot of my outbursts in here, because I have been quite bad, of late, just crying and I didn't want to take part in anything, and I've told the staff now I made excuses that, for not going to OT, I could have been there I just didn't want to go, and I said I wasn't well enough and I've been, and it's so annoying then when I hear other people, not to mention any, patients' names but, you must know the one I mean, going on and on about his past, I, I feel sorry for him, John, I mean, you have met him, I've heard this story dozens of t-, you hear it half past eleven at night, seven o'clock in the morning, goes back to when he was nineteen, if I went back to when I was nineteen, it wouldna paint a very pre-, pretty picture either probably, but it's nothing to do why, with why I'm in here. That, I admit he's, he's got nothing left, but he's still got time to, make a life for himself I think, think he quite likes it here (laughs).'

Through such social processes of interaction and moral reasoning (*cf.* McHugh's (1968) account of deviance) patients participated in, and in some cases resisted, the construction of their own and each other's deviance. Informal accounting was thus one vehicle for construction of – or challenges to – the ascription of mental illness (*cf.* Smith 1978).

Accounting for practice and nursing research

Previous nursing research has taken for granted that nurses' accounts in the systems of accounting organized for their practical interests can be considered unproblematically from a theoretical perspective. If nurses in practice do not 'pick up' what the researcher thinks is of theoretical interest, they are considered inadequate.

To understand practitioners' accountability *vis à vis* researchers it is important to recognize that there are two orders of accounting in nursing research: nurses' and patients' accounts (designed for their practical purposes) are represented in the researcher's accounting system, e.g. in a theoretical account. Nursing researchers' theoretical accounts typically fail to consider the nature of practical accounting. Accounting by nurses in psychiatric admission wards is systematically organized for the production of a form of social reality, i.e. the ward at the time. Nurses have an interest in knowing and being able to report how the ward is, what the main things to be noted are, and so on. Researchers accounting for nursing practice should therefore be reflexive. The researcher establishing a system of accounting based on some interest (whether the researcher's interest or the putative interests of the researched), and trying to enrol nurses and patients in it, faces problems of concealment and other forms of resistance.

Templates for accounting

Templates for accounting in psychiatric nursing include, for example, the system of case recording and communication outlined by Marks *et al.* (1977) as the basis for the work of nurse behavioural psychotherapists. This includes documentation of screening, assessment, treatment and measurement, follow-up, and reporting to the referral source. A second example is the documentation, based on Falloon's work, used by Brooker (1990) for family management of schizophrenia.

A template for sequential accounts was found by Tilley (1995). Patients sometimes indicated that their ability to give an account of themselves was dependent on the nurses having first given an account to them. Nurses' accounts provided 'templates' which the patients could use to structure their own accounts. Some patients noted that nurses gave accounts on their behalf when they could not account for themselves,[9] thereby assuming responsibility for the patient until the patient was able to account for herself or himself.

The relationship between nurse and patient was mirrored in the formal relationship between their accounts: the relationship and the accounts were 'symbiotic'[10] (*cf.* Shotter 1984; Harré, 1983). Thus, a patient said:

> '**Patient:** See some ones'll say to (? you), 'What's wrong with you you're no looking so well?', or, 'You're maybe looking better this morning', you know, and you feel, Well, maybe I am a wee bit better, and, cos, some of the nurses here have said to me, over the last week, I have improved, and I know I have improved myself, over the last week....'

Through these processes the patient as a person was symbolically constructed through accounting. In the process, the nurses noticed the patient. As a patient said: 'And, you feel that, it is being taken notice of, you know, you're no just sitting there as a lump. And, you're being watched, but, in a, the nicest way'. Having noticed, the nurses provided accounts of the patient and to her, accounts that enabled her to be understood and to understand herself as 'mentally ill'. They interpreted her as a kind of person – not a lump, but a person who was ill – and took what was seen as 'the right attitude' toward her. In a symbiotic account the patient was provided with an understanding of the kind of person she was, as well as an understanding of why she was here and what she had to do. She was someone who had been mentally ill and was recovering. The symbolic construction of the patient as ill was sustained through the system of accounts (including symbiotic accounts) and accountability within a moral order. Symbiotic accounting was, in this sense, resocialization or 'therapy' in practice (*cf*. Berger and Luckmann 1967).

ACCOUNTABILITY

A useful working definition of accountability can be found in Thompson *et al.* (1994). The term implies an ability to give an account and a responsibility to tell others what has been done. With regard to work, the latter sense includes both nurses' obligation to provide accounts to managers and doctors, and patients' obligations to provide accounts to nurses. Accountability, considered as readiness and obligation to give an account, can be construed from theoretical, organizational, professional and practical (disciplinary) perspectives.

If accounts relate more to knowledge, and accounting to systems of power, accountability relates to moral order. Accounts are devices and occasions for discipline: opening one to surveillance, to judgement of normality, to interpretation and to correction. Accounting is a form of discipline – a process of confession and response. Accountability refers to the rights and obligations entailed by participation in a system of accounts and the norms related to the system of accounting. It involves taking one's place in a system of accounting, becoming the 'I' in documents circulated to 'them'.

The counterpart to formal and informal accounts and systems of accounting is formal and informal accountability. Nurses as accountable practitioners can be seen as 'Janus-faced'. Janus, the deity associated with openings, is an apt emblem for nurses who have to keep patients 'open' as accountable subjects in wards or in the community; to keep open the possibilities of exchange between hospital and community; and to act as gatekeepers in systems of need and resource determination. Janus had two faces, one facing in, the other out. Psychiatric nurses are accountable to the wider community of which they and patients are members, the community knit together by common sense. They are also accountable to professional and institutional bodies requiring them to be ready and willing to provide accounts legitimated by reference to law, theory, codes of conduct or procedure manuals. Janus-faced accountability – implying accountability to managers and the profession as well as responsibility to the patient in face-to-face interaction[11] - is, for practical purposes, the essential characteristic of psychiatric nursing.

Nurses are most fundamentally accountable to the others – nurses and patients – with whom they share the 'paramount reality' and morality of day-to-day life of the ward or community. Other systems of accountability, e.g. theoretical, research, legal and professional, are both superimposed on and depend on this. The dual aspect of nurses' accountability in the wards is conveyed by the term 'savvy', used by a charge nurse to describe what was needed in someone who was to nurse in his ward. 'Savvy' was the knowledge needed to work in the ward, including the knowledge that staff nurses should manage the paperwork – the formal mechanism of accountability – so that the charge nurse was free to manage the informal system of accountability, the sense of the coherence between the day-to-day life in the ward and 'my (i.e. the charge nurse's) reality'. The charge nurse picked up the latter sense in face-to-face contact and talk with the patients. 'Savvy' was necessary for cooperative work geared toward accountably handing over the ward (or, by extension, the community psychiatric nurse's patch) to the next shift.

Psychiatric nurses' legal accountability and the Mental Health Act (1983 [Scotland 1984])

To some extent, psychiatric nurses' accountability, like that of other nurses, is determined by registration. This accountability encompasses issues related to professional conduct, maintaining competence to practise, record keeping, ensuring informed consent to treatment, advocacy and confidentiality. These more general issues will not be reviewed here.

More specific powers, responsibility and accountability in terms of the law, devolve on the first-level Registered Mental Nurse under the terms of the Mental Health Act (1983 [Scotland, 1984]). Ritter (1992), and more fully in Ritter (in press), summarizes these aspects:

> 'The nurses' six-hour holding power was another major innovation of the Mental Health Act (1983). The power to detain a patient in hospital for up to six hours is one which the nurse exercises as part of his or her professional judgement as to the need to restrain a person from leaving hospital. Although the detention period lasts only until a doctor can assess the patient, or for six hours, whichever is shorter, no doctor of other member of staff can order the nurse to exercise the holding power. In this way the Mental Health Act 1983 recognizes the professional autonomy of psychiatric nurses and registered mental handicap nurses.'

The reader interested in the legal aspects of psychiatric nurses' accountability in relation to this Act is referred to Bluglass (1983), Unsworth (1987), and Jones (1985).

Earlier in this chapter, the questions were raised: What understanding of 'account' is useful for interpreting psychiatric nursing? What is the paradigm of the legitimate account in practice and in researchers' discourse on practice? How do nurses hear accounts, including explanations, stories and excuses, as practically useful in the work of, for example, admission wards? It was argued that it is useful to regard accounts as methods for 'smoothing rough passages in social life' (Harré 1979). Nurses and patients who encounter each other during rough passages need a common sense of what a legitimate account is, when one is required and who may require one. This understanding implies that one thing a nurse might do for a patient is to help her or him account in order to smooth a rough passage. This involves a double kind of responsibility: the nurse, on behalf of the patient, taking the responsibility for providing an account of illness, problem or ordinary social life by means of which the patient claims or disclaims responsibility for what occasioned the 'rough passage'.

Management of accountability

The author (Tilley 1995) concluded that patients and nurses are interdependent in their accomplishment of accountability. Their accountability is not an attribute of nurse or patient; rather, it is a social construct, the reality of which is negotiated in face-to-face interaction.

Nurses' and patients' interdependence as accountable subjects is fundamentally rooted in the morality and accountability of everyday life, drawing on it and reproducing it (*cf.* Giddens 1976). In psychiatric nurse–patient interaction, everyday life and the selves of nurse and patient are produced, reproduced and, where necessary, negotiated. This point may be clarified by an example. The production of knowledge of self is seen in a student nurse's account:

'**Nurse:** I remember talking to Patient 8 at, eh, the OT, when we had to, write these things down about ourselves, and I said that I felt she had never opened up to me, that I enjoyed her conversation, but I felt that she was hiding something. And she denied it. (? Uh eh), quite annoyed, 'Oh no, I, I've told you everything, Shula, I don't know what I need to tell you'. (Note: N's voice is a 'mock innocent' voice.) But then, she came to me later and said that she had a friend up, and she had been telling her, what I had said. And the friend that's known her frae, childhood, had said that she had the same impression of Patient 8, that she always held back, and didna give all herself, em, was a wee bit reserved. And Patient 8 hadnae felt that at all. So, I was a bit annoyed, cos I says 'Patient 8, I hope I didnae embarrass you, or offend you', and she says 'No, no', but she says 'It's just interesting what other people think', and she says 'I don't think I'm reserved'. But she says 'Both you and my friend have said that, so,' she says 'maybe I am'...Cos she said that she never thought that she was a wee bit private. But she says 'When both of you is, under that impression', she says, 'maybe I am, maybe I am a wee bit reserved'.'

The patient's interpretation of the nurse's action suggests the relevance of Foucault's (1982) analysis of 'pastoral power'. Self-interpretation and other-interpretation are practices through which the patient takes part in the production of truth about herself. Through an individualizing discourse, she comes to know herself and is known as the kind of individual she is.[12]

Identity as the subject/object of knowledge is constituted by or in relation to (in resistance to) a discourse which operates as 'knowledge/power' (Foucault 1982). Accounts then are 'ways a human being turns him or herself into a subject' in Foucault's (1982) double-edged sense of 'subject', i.e. 'subject to someone else by control or dependence, and tied to his own identity by a conscience or self-knowledge'.

In giving a first-person account, the individual – patient or nurse – subjects herself or himself to the moral order in which such an account is required, to the truth of the account, and to the one who requires the account. This argument echoes Altschul's (1972) view that the systems of accountability and accounting in which psychiatric nurses participate with patients are systems of social control.

The empirical evidence cited in this chapter (based on Tilley 1995) indicates that psychiatric nurses and patients are asymmetrically interdependent in the work of management of accountability – that is, in relations of power. Nurses could command the appearance of the patient as an accountable subject more readily than the patients could command the appearance of the nurses. Nurses' power to play their part in their place of work depends on their ability to get accounts from patients, hence on their ability to manage the patients' accountability.[13] The nurses' work can thus be regarded as a form of disciplinary power (Foucault 1979):

'Disciplinary power...is exercised through its invisibility; at the same time it imposes on those whom it subjects a principle of compulsory visibility. In discipline, it is the subjects who have to be seen.'

In this chapter the focus has been on the nurses' and patients' accomplishment of visibility through a discourse in which patients were construed as 'presenting' the features which, in nurses' accounts, characterized them as patients (cf. Atkinson 1977).

Limiting accountability in practice

Part of nurses' competent management of accountability is competence in limiting it. They accomplish this in various ways. Accountability is closely linked with the use of pronouns. Nurses in practice (Tilley 1995) could claim and disclaim accountability by using 'we' rather than 'I':

> '**Nurse:** ...Well in a way, the kind of conversation almost got to the point of...discharge,...I was kinda sorta saying to her I think this explains your illness...I think this explains why you're the way you are. And I think I probably, I may have used the term 'we'...We think this is what's happened to you, this is why we want to put you on the stat-, back to status quo. You know, so it's almost talking to someone as if they're just leaving that they're having everything explained to them...what's happened.
> **Researcher:** Right, right, right, right.
> **Nurse:** '(?) this is our opinion'. It's like when you know the surgeon says 'Goodbye' to you after taking your appendix out....'

The use of pronouns indicates features of the moral order. The nurse's use of 'we' can be regarded as legitimating their acting in a role which was usually reserved for doctors. Pronoun use could occasion work on the person as well as resistance to that work, for example when nurses challenged a patient's claim that (the patient as) 'I' could not do something. Command of the discourse thus had a counterpart in command of the person. The nurses managed the appearance of, and socially constructed, both themselves and patients as accountable subjects.[14]

Nurses may also practise limiting accountability through self-management in the formal systems of accountability, that is, by managing their own appearances as accountable subjects in written records. This limiting of accountability may be learned in practice. Thus, students (Tilley 1995) were told to write 'facts not impressions' in their entries for the nursing Kardex (the daily written record). The nurses excluded ('managed out') from written records interpretations which might have been relevant to – indeed, might have mediated – their practice of power in interaction. Nurses also limited accountability through subscription to an understanding about individual style and the grounds of action. According to this understanding, each nurse was an individual; each individual nurse had his or her own style; and any given nurse might pick up more in a given situation than would another nurse, and hence would handle things differently (*cf.* Pollock 1989). This understanding legitimated a general account to the effect that different nurses would do things differently, as well as a corollary that a nurse could not be expected to account for another nurse's actions. Additionally, nurses limited their accountability by working on the basis of an understanding that interpretation, rhetorical skill, style and character – all necessary for their work – were conveyed in talk, not writing. Indeed, the nurses' practical accountability was founded on and grounded in an oral discourse. Their practices reflexively maintained the primacy of talk in practice, the foundation of psychiatric nurses' oral culture (*cf.* Grypdonk 1987).

Templates for the accountable psychiatric nurse

One template of accountability in the psychiatric nursing literature is the model of the nurse as personal scientist (Barker 1982). The nurse is represented as a reflexive, self-monitoring person who attempts to meet the needs of a patient or client ethically by practice based quasi single-case experimental design. Another model (Reynolds and Cormack 1982) is the theoretically guided, diagnostically informed nurse. A third (Brooker 1990) is the nurse who recognizes the primacy of the needs of the most severely ill and the obligation to help them by managing resources effectively and efficiently.

The currently available models for accountable psychiatric nursing share certain features. They are rational and informed by a version of scientific method based on the benchmark of experimental design. They locate the accountable nurse through a discourse on care and/or therapy, linked with a discourse on interprofessional distinctions and the need for nurses to establish their domains of competence *vis à vis* psychiatrists or social workers.

CONCLUSION

Both formal and informal aspects of psychiatric nurses' accountability are related to wider debates and struggles over what constitutes a legitimate account, a legitimate system of accounting, and accountability. Psychiatric nursing 'territories', marked by discourses of research, theory, practice and management, are currently being constructed and defended. In these territories, structured by human labour, including interpretation, authority is legitimated and power is enacted through processes of accounting addressed to and addressing, locating, 'hailing' (*cf.* Althusser 1971) accountable moral beings. The argument of this chapter is that appropriate working understandings of 'account', 'accounting' and 'accountability' can be developed by reference to empirical data and to the interpretative, commonsense practicalities of day-to-day practice. Recognition of two essential aspects of psychiatric nurses' practice – the Janus-faced character of their accountability, and their interdependence with patients in the management of that accountability – could usefully inform a practical curriculum for the education of psychiatric nurses.

NOTES

1 A problem with previous nursing research is that it treated accounts as if they were meant to be theorizings, interpretable in terms of scientific rationality (see Schuetz 1943).

2 The role of accounts in legitimation can be seen in studies of deviance construction, largely within the symbolic interactionist tradition (Scheff 1966; McHugh 1968; Rubington and Weinberg 1987).

3 The claim that responsibility is established through diagnosis (or through 'objective' testing: see MacIlwaine 1980) can be challenged in two respects: diagnosis may follow from successful attribution of responsibility or non-responsibility (*cf.* May and

Kelly 1982; Tilley 1995); and the practical meaning of diagnosis depends on the interpretation of the diagnosis in the practice setting.

4 For discussions of how practice ideologies articulate with practices of need assessment see Smith (1980) on ideologies in social work; and Towell (1975) and Pollock (1989) on psychiatric nursing ideologies.

5 By 'it' may be meant the problem, the illness or an otherwise defined focus of defined work.

6 The nurses resisted patients' attempts to impose a service role on them. Injunctions not to treat the sites like hotels or holiday camps served this function, as did disparagement of 'bed and breakfast' patients (who were admitted by duty doctors on Friday nights and discharged on Monday mornings). They resisted it most strongly through expressing the ideology of work and responsibility.

7 The first nurse's discourse can be read as an account of the patient's resistance to the nurses' 'pastoral power' (Foucault 1982), through which she would have been subjected, or subjected herself, to the truth of herself as an individual.

8 The present author's research in progress shows that psychiatric nurses sometimes resist the formal systems of accounting and operate alternative systems. Thus, nurses might resist assessing patients to put them on a waiting list, on the grounds that relief of the bureaucratic manager's responsibility (the responsibility for ensuring that patients are seen) is accomplished at the expense of the practitioner who, having seen and heard the patient, incurs an obligation to respond, an obligation which she or he cannot fulfil.

9 I observed this in the case of accounts given to excuse patients who were psychotic. Accounts for non-responsibility were given for such patients ('she doesn't know herself').

10 Symbiotic relationships are essential to the development of persons. In a symbiotic relationship one learns what one is doing through the accounts given by another (Harré 1983; Shotter 1984).

11 Desmond Ryan (seminar, Edinburgh University, 1993) is developing i) a concept of the 'amphibian nurse', who has to survive in different elements; and ii) distinctions between responsibility and accountability useful for nurses.

12 See Foucault (1982) on 'pastoral power'. The 'recovery of strays' to a 'paramount reality', may be interpreted as a form of pastoral power.

13 Nurses and patients are interdependent in that the authority of each depends on legitimation by the other (cf. May and Kelly 1982).

14 Peplau (1952) understood that claims of agency related to patients' use of pronouns to claim or deny agency ('I', 'we'). My analysis suggests a further development of Peplau's insight: namely, that by claiming the patient-as-subject ('I' in the patient's discourse) as subject (topic in the nurse's discourse), the nurse managed the appearance of himself as an accountable subject. He did so by managing the appearance of the patient through command of the discourse. See also Pollock (1989) on psychiatric nurses' management of appearances.

Accountability in community nursing | 8

Sarah Baggaley and Alison Bryans

INTRODUCTION

A wide range of meanings have been attributed to the concept of community. Core ideas generally have a positive tone, and include notions of interdependence or connectedness and belonging, rather than mere proximity or simply sharing physical space. As one author puts it: 'People are part of their whole surroundings, like cells in a single body' (Seedhouse 1986).

The concept of community also shares the complexity and sophistication of a single body and its dynamic nature. What, therefore, is the relevance of these meanings to nurses working in the community? First, it is necessary for community nurses who wish to be successful in their practice to seek to understand and embrace the character of the community in which they work, and the significance of this for its inhabitants. This involves awareness of the total environment, a working knowledge of a social model of health (Williams *et al.* 1993), and a flexible and holistic approach to health care, rather than too narrow a focus. Secondly, the working environment is filled with a vast array of other workers with whom the community nurse must cooperate in order to achieve the best deal for clients. Special skills in networking (which include the identification and use of available resources) are essential, as well as good interpersonal skills. Thirdly, as well as being accountable to individual clients, to line management and to the UKCC (United Kingdom Central Council for Nursing, Midwifery and Health Visiting) (Watson 1992), the community nurse may be said to have a particular responsibility towards the community itself.

Some of these issues will be explored in greater depth in this chapter, particularly when discussing the legal and moral aspects of accountability in the community.

ORGANIZATIONAL ISSUES AFFECTING THE ACCOUNTABILITY OF COMMUNITY NURSES

The recent wave of NHS reforms has created considerable challenges for community nursing: boundaries are shifting and the future is unclear. However, in order to set the scene within which community nurses are expected to be accountable for their practice, organizational issues within primary health care which have certain implications for accountability in nursing practice in the community will be discussed briefly.

The dominant themes of the NHS reforms which are currently being implemented include increasing preventive activities and extending the role of primary care. Many community nurses have probably welcomed the shift in emphasis away from secondary care. After all, the acute sector has long enjoyed the lion's share of resources and the higher profile, as biomedicine advances. Now, perhaps, community 'frontline' services will have their day, as the World Health Organization (WHO) advocated in 1978 in the Alma Ata Declaration; this was accepted in principle by the UK government, which clearly identified primary health care as the key to health for all (WHO 1978).

However, a certain dissonance is now apparent between current government policies aimed at creating a healthier nation and action strategies developed by the WHO since Alma Ata to meet European health targets. The latter have a distinct community development/public health focus, citing the key areas of 'health promotion action' as building healthy public policy, creating supportive environments, strengthening community action, developing personal skills and reorientating health services (WHO 1986). UK government policies go some way in this direction, and The Health of the Nation initiative is to be monitored by a Cabinet committee, with representation from 11 government departments (DoH 1992b), indicating growing awareness of the need for intersectoral working. However, the greatest emphasis by far has been on seeking to change people's health behaviours, primarily through screening and professional advice.

The leading role of the GP has been a major component of recent reforms, evidenced by the new GP contract (DoH 1990c), and has obvious implications for the autonomy of community nurses and their public health role in the future (Billingham 1991; Potrykus 1993). One consequence of the recent reforms of general practice is that community nurses are cast in the role of providers, whose care is purchased by GP fundholding practices (NHSME 1993). This is part and parcel of the introduction of market principles to the health-care sector. Since the priorities of the particular practice are liable to prevail in the context of this purchaser–provider relationship, concerns have been expressed by the health visiting profession regarding the potential demise of primary prevention in favour of secondary screening. Calnan and others point out that

> '...health care reforms, although recognizing the role of community nurses...(make the) assumption that GPs will be the leaders. That is to say,

health promotion will become GP-centric, which is contrary to WHO directives which emphasize the crucial role of nurses' (Williams *et al.* 1993).

Concern has also been expressed by a variety of professionals, including a standing committee of the British Medical Association (BMA), that the greater purchasing powers of fundholders may erode the public health function of health visitors (Beecham 1992; Barker 1993; Orr 1993; Potrykus 1993).

On the positive side, there is the potential for fundholding practices to raise the profile of primary health care and to develop more effective working relationships with the full range of community nurses who may be involved with their practice populations. It is fair to suggest that some practices could make better use of the expertise of nurse specialists, such as community psychiatric nurses and community mental handicap nurses, whose services are currently underused (Naughton 1993).

It is also arguable whether decision making about community nursing should be the preserve of either general practitioners or of managers whose occupational background is in neither nursing nor medicine. Huntingdon (1993) states that the purchaser–provider split further reinforces the confinement of nursing to 'operational, rather than strategic, roles and functions', a confinement implicit in the introduction of general management to the NHS in 1983. She argues that the nursing profession should pursue quality for service users by involving itself in strategic planning, where such central issues as effectiveness, equity and efficiency are at stake. These issues are close relations to autonomy and accountability, and cannot be left to those outside community nursing if nurses working in community settings are to be accountable in any real sense.

There are options to the 'GP-centric' model which do not appear to have received due consideration. For instance, Barker (1993) has suggested that health visitors should function either as practice health visitors (employed directly by GPs) or as community health visitors, employed by public health directorates. It will be interesting to see how such organizational issues will be resolved in the longer term, and how involved at management level community nurses actually become.

A further aspect of recent reforms which is linked to these issues is the potential for greater patient participation in both planning and the delivery of care. This notion is already inherent in the values of community nursing and is one to which we will consequently return later in the chapter.

CURRENT ISSUES IN COMMUNITY NURSING

Changes in the organization of primary care, coupled with reforms in nurse education, have resulted in considerable anxiety and uncertainty regarding the future of community nursing. Much of the current debate centres upon the issues of resource allocation and skill mix.

Resource allocation and skill mix

These questions are central to the present call for a systematic approach to setting staffing levels among health visitors and district nurses. It would be highly appropriate if the health needs of the population were seen to be leading employment issues. This would increase the accountability of a profession which is providing the service, by justifying its practice to both the public that it serves and to its health service managers, who are the purchasers. However, the current fear among staff is that the driving force behind the present scrutiny is concerned less with improving the service delivered and is more of a cost-cutting exercise.

The issue of cost cannot be ignored in any discussion on accountability, as wastage of resources is obviously not in the public interest. Job dissatisfaction concerning administration among community nurses is marked (Wade 1993). The growing amount of time spent on administrative matters was particularly highlighted by health visitors and, to a lesser extent, by district nurses. Frustration stemmed from the feeling that nursing skills are best deployed with clients or patients. Wade states in her conclusion:

'It is clearly not cost effective if highly qualified staff spend a dispropor-tionate time doing clerical work. This is a matter which requires urgent clarification as it suggests that the focus for skill-mix review should be administrative rather than clinical.'

The NHSME (1993) review proposes that £40m a year could be saved by halv-ing the numbers of 'G' grade district nurses and replacing them with less quali-fied or untrained staff – cuts that can apparently be simply achieved through a simple, crude task analysis. The swift combined response by the professional bodies, the District Nurses' Association (DNA) and the Health Visitors' Association (HVA) (Anonymous 1992), stated that this would seriously under-mine the government's attempt to further consumer interests by expanding and improving community services, as set out in *The Patient's Charter* (DoH 1991a) and *Caring for People* (1990a).

Cowley (1993) demonstrates that the NHSME review is based on flawed beliefs regarding the simplicity of nursing practice. She feels that it ignores the need for professional judgement, the variety of skills and the level of decision making in continuing assessment and practice. The key issue is not to confuse grade mix with skill mix: the former is concerned with grades, their costs and their activities, whereas the latter 'allows a clear and necessary link to be made between needs, skills and outcomes' (Cowley 1993).

If the complexity of nursing practice in the community is to be better under-stood, then one of the priorities is for nurses to explain how skills, decisions and outcomes are related. This ability to articulate clearly is one of the concepts at the core of accountability.

Batey and Lewis (1982) cited in the Royal College of Nursing *Health Visitors' Advisory Group Document* (RCN 1984) states that accountability is 'the fulfilment of a formal obligation to disclose to others the purpose, principles, procedures, relationships, results, income and expenditures for which one has authority'. Such disclosure can also be of positive service to nurses. There has never been more need to convince not only client groups of the benefits of the service, but also managers who may not have a nursing background, and purchasers, be they GPs or health authorities/health boards, and other allied professions.

Health visitors in particular suffer from a lack of recognition about what they do and are therefore inclined towards a feeling of professional vulnerability. Much of their work in health promotion, prevention and support is felt to be implicit and therefore not clearly demonstrable. An ability to make skills and professional judgement visible and explicit, and to demonstrate which outcomes have been achieved, could convince others of their worth as well as enhancing accountability.

Recognition of the specific expertise of different types of community nurse becomes particularly important when some duties must be delegated to others of a different grade. *The Scope of Professional Practice* (UKCC 1992b) states in clauses 9.5 and 9.6 that:

'The registered nurse, midwife or health visitor must recognize and honour the direct or indirect personal accountability borne for all aspects of professional practice and must, in serving the interests of patients and clients and the wider interests of society, avoid any inappropriate delegation to others which compromises those interests.'

Some of the arguments and concerns felt have been discussed, but there are already clear indications that both district nurses and health visitors will lead teams of staff nurses and support workers. The appearance of the Project 2000 nurse will hasten this development. To some extent district nurses have experience of heading teams, but health visitors less so.

The concern with managerial accountability becomes evident when considering appropriate areas for delegation, as indicated above, by the UKCC. Clear decisions have to be made as to which patients and clients require direct care from the health visitor and district nurse. In some ways, however, this can be seen to be promoting an area which district nurses and health visitors feel is one of their special skills, that of assessment.

The future position of the Project 2000 nurse in the community is proving to be a thorny issue for many. Some managers envisage this leading to a reduction in highly skilled community staff. The range of what managers expect such nurses will be undertaking in the community is diverse, from being supervised at all times with no caseload to directly replacing district nurses and health visitors. The change in the philosophy and content of education in the P2000 programme, with the student gaining continuing experience in the community and hospital settings, means that the first-level nurse could be used in community nursing when linked with the experience and decision-making skills of the district nurse and health visitor.

Twinn raises the issue of relationship difficulties between nurses of different disciplines that Cumberlege (DHSS 1986) identified. These can only be detrimental to standards of client care, and Twinn (1991) emphasizes that 'teamwork requires respect for the practice of other practitioners'.

The increased numbers of students and the lengthier time that they are out on community placements also poses issues for accountability. Orr (1993) feels strongly that they are not in the community to learn to be health visitors and district nurses, and identifies a lack of clarity about the purpose of the community placement and the unrealistic expectations of what they are likely to achieve. Greater thought about the preparation for individual practitioners responsible for organizing placements is necessary. There are also issues of accountability concerning clients as well: clients need to clearly understand the role of the student and have access to qualified members of staff. Clients are generally willing to participate in students' learning but, to date, have not been exposed to the anticipated numbers within their own homes. Qualified staff must not compromise levels of care in trying to accommodate the learning needs of students.

Profiling need and evaluating outcomes

Lightfoot et al. (1992), in their research into the deployment of community nurses, indicated the following areas as needing a more systematic approach:

- assessment and prioritization of the community nursing needs of the local population;
- development of appropriate measures of service outcomes;
- definition of the roles of district nursing and health visiting services.

Currently, one of the clearest ways in which community nurses are trying to address the first area is by health profiling. This can be at community/locality or practice level for those nurses who are attached to GP practices.

Which data and who will collect them has to be established before a profile can be compiled. This needs to be negotiated at the outset by the practitioners and managers involved. Blackburn (1992) argues that poverty should be an integral part of every health profile. Possible criteria for inclusion are suggested by Twinn et al. (1990), but these should vary according to local needs and circumstances. Following analysis, it should be possible to establish the health needs of the defined population so that appropriate objectives can be set. The need for practitioners and management to recognize and document unmet needs and alert the appropriate authorities is seen by Twinn et al. as being important in terms of professional accountability and the professional code of conduct. Profiles, as demonstrated by Hugman and McCready (1993), can be a useful tool when setting standards and considering audit, which will be described more fully later.

A discussion of the ways of finding sound methods and instruments for evaluating outcomes is not within the scope of this chapter. It is certainly an area that has exercised many authors and generated much debate. For instance, Chalmers' (1993) study was undertaken as she identified that 'there is little empirically based knowledge of how health visitors carry out these functions [searching out and stimulating client's awareness of health needs] in their daily work'. Her study does indicate that many health visitors were able to uncover health needs through their daily work.

Increasingly there are examples of ways in which this is being achieved in what is an area that needs further development: Holden *et al.*'s (1989) controlled study of the effectiveness of counselling postnatally depressed women is one, and Barker and Anderson's (1988) work on the development of a child surveillance programme is another.

The community care aspect of the NHS and Community Care Act of 1990 (DoH 1990b) was eventually implemented in April 1993. One of the aims was to move from being service driven to being needs driven so that clients should have a greater say in what they would like and in what they feel they need.

Community nurses have a major role to play following the implementation of the Community Care Act owing to the increased number of vulnerable people in the community. District nurses, in particular, are finding their workload increased in terms of assessment, coordination and service provision. Included in the policy changes was the requirement for local authorities to become the leading agencies for care in the community, acting as purchasers. Salter and Salter (1993) noted that this has produced a paradoxical situation where responsibility for a highly complex piece of social policy legislation is carried by bodies over which the DoH has no control, despite retaining national responsibility for community care.

The changes have fostered a multidisciplinary approach such that social service departments and health authorities/boards have been required to work out agreements for the provision of integrated care. There have been difficulties in defining the difference between social and health care, and therefore who is the best person to provide that care (Healey 1993). Many authorities insist that they have not been allocated enough funding to meet the raised public expectation that comprehensive social and health care will be provided. Where there is a shortfall there is often a greater pressure to rely more heavily on community nurses, since they are not funded by the authorities. There is no evidence of greater numbers of community nursing staff, therefore in many areas nurses are having to find the balance between the patients' needs and wishes and what resources are available within the health and social service budgets. Accountability to their clients can be increasingly difficult for nurses, given the different cultures, structures and ways of accountability to management of the agencies with whom the nurse may be trying to liaise (Hunter 1993).

Legal and professional issues in community nursing

Nurses have been attracted to working in the community for a variety of reasons, but high on the list is the feeling that they have greater autonomy and professional responsibility, allowing for more freedom in their decision making and the care they provide. Indeed, the recent moves (*Patient's Charter* DoH 1992a) to enable each patient to have a named nurse is not a new concept in the community. However, as many authors (Bergman 1981; Batey and Lewis 1982a; RCN 1984; McLymont *et al.* (1986) indicate, responsibility can only be a reality if the professional has the authority to act. Clearly, the authority is invested in community nurses for much of their practice through education and knowledge but, as McClymont *et al.* point out, 'responsibility without authority undermines professional autonomy and creates frustration'.

An example of where there can be problems is if a district nurse or health visitor assesses that an individual needs a variety of services but the authority to provide them is outside their jurisdiction. An elderly person might be assessed as needing assistance in the home or requiring aids and adaptations, but such resources are in the control of social service departments. The implementation of the Community Care Act, with greater control of resources being put into the hands of social service departments, has highlighted such issues and caused concern for many community nurses.

Independent professional practice, as valued by community nurses, brings with it a greater responsibility to have the highest standards of professional competence. The risk of failure to deliver optimum care can be greater when individuals have a greater degree of autonomy.

Responsibility is inextricably linked with accountability. This is the key to ensuring that greater autonomy for decision making and practice coincides with good standards of care. Greater freedom for the individual nurse brings with it the necessity for enhanced personal or moral accountability and integrity, rather than relying on externally imposed control. This area will be discussed more fully later.

Professional responsibility means that there is an accountability to the profession as a whole, and thus to society. In the case of nursing it is the UKCC which has a mandatory function through the Nurses, Midwives and Health Visitors Act (1979) to advise its practitioners on standards of professional conduct. In a formal way it does so by registering practitioners and by a variety of published codes. It is the duty of every nurse to be totally conversant with the standards of care and scope of professional practice laid down by the UKCC.

Various UKCC documents, such as *The Code of Professional Conduct* (1992a), *The Scope of Professional Practice* (1992b) and *Exercising Accountability* (1989) clearly state that all nurses are personally accountable for their own practice. It is made explicit that it is not only activities but also omissions for which they can be held accountable.

Team work

The majority of community nurses work within teams, whether it be the primary health-care team or within a team of nurses. Without doubt, individual and family needs are often too complex to be met by one profession. Multidisciplinary teams function well and provide the opportunity to bring together a variety of skills and professional competencies, so that more comprehensive care can be provided.

Precisely where accountability lies within the context of team care can sometimes be the least considered issue. Rowden (1987), contemplating his time spent representing nurses in inquiries, hearings and tribunals, observes that 'problems often arise because nurses practise under the misguided belief that someone else will answer for actions taken by the individual nurse'. Health visitors, who are increasingly undertaking the practice of giving immunizations to babies and young children, should be quite clear in their own minds that, despite the fact that GPs often put their names to the immunization forms, in order to ensure payment under the GP contract, it is the health visitor who will be held accountable for both the advice and the immunization given. It is therefore in their own interests to be fully confident in their own abilities before undertaking such work. The RCN document *Accountability in Health Visiting* (1984) also states that 'team accountability can never override the accountability of the individual nurse for her own professional decisions and actions', also noting that professionals cannot be held accountable for the actions and practice of other members of the team.

Preparation for practice in the community

It is clear that a sound knowledge base and competencies are prerequisites for practice. Given that nurses are held accountable, they should be aware of their limitations and decline to perform actions unless they are able to do so appropriately. Current and potential changes planned for nurses in the community have highlighted these issues.

Since the implementation of the GP contract in 1990 there has been a great increase in the numbers of practice nurses, estimated to exceed 10 000 (Audit Commission 1992). Most of these are directly employed by GPs. There is an enormous variation in practice nurses' educational backgrounds (Wade 1993; Thurtle 1993), which has led to worries, not least by the nurses themselves, that many are inadequately prepared for the role that they are expected by GPs to fulfil (Peachey 1992; Goodwin *et al.* 1991). Some are still working without job descriptions or protocols, with all the implications this has for lack of professional accountability (Paterson 1993). Stilwell (1991) argues that practice nurses should become more assertive about what they consider is appropriate for them to be doing in general practice, which might mean becoming more involved in drawing up practice protocols.

Cumberlege (DHSS 1986) was one of the first to point out the lack of appropriate training for practice nurses. Their needs are now being considered to a greater extent, with many more courses becoming available; however, provision is still patchy and such courses are not mandatory. The UKCC's *Scope of Professional Practice* (1992b) concludes that 'Any local arrangements must ensure that registered nurses, midwives and health visitors are assisted to undertake and are enabled to fulfil any suitable adjustments to their scope of practice'. This must surely include the availability of educational provision as well as addressing the issues of study time and replacement cover for practice nurses.

Future changes that will have an impact upon district nurses and health visitors include nurse prescribing, which passed its last stages in parliament in 1992. While and Rees (1993), in their small questionnaire survey, found that district nurses, in general, welcomed the prospect of being able to prescribe; health visitors were less enthusiastic. A detailed knowledge of products used, based on research findings, is necessary for nurses to be fully accountable to their patients and to their professional body, as they will be responsible for prescribing such treatments in the future. The Advisory Group on Nurse Prescribing suggested that practical, pharmacological and therapeutic aspects be included in an educational package in order to augment the existing knowledge base of district nurses and health visitors. From the results of their survey, While and Rees (1993) suggest that the existing knowledge base for prescribing is patchy. A wider programme is required, including aspects of diagnosis, enhanced knowledge of products, and an understanding of the accountability, professional responsibility and legal requirements fundamental to nurse prescribing.

Nurse prescribing is a specific example of future developments. At the time of writing there are also wider issues under consideration, such as the role of Project 2000 diplomates in the community, as discussed earlier. Their role is clearly linked to the UKCC's finalized details of its post-registration education and practice (PREP), which now includes community nursing. The future educational requirements for community nurses will be different from the present, given the changing requirements and expectations and taking into account the P2000 nurses' experience. The publication of the PREP proposals caused major debate among professionals which will continue for some time, but the requirement for nurses to maintain and update their professional skills has been universally welcomed. In the future, nurses will be required to give evidence that they are doing so, thus fulfilling their obligations under the professional code. This emphasizes that the individual is accountable to the professional body for maintaining and developing their professional skills and expertise. There is, however, unease that employers may take the minimum 5 study days requirement over 3 years as being the standard requirement.

Among other changes proposed in the reforms are the post-registration levels of community nurses. 'Advanced practitioner' appears to incorporate some of the managerial role of the current line managers, but seems to envisage the concept of clinical management closer to that outlined in the Cumberlege Report. Responsibilities indicated include monitoring and improving standards of care through the supervision of practice; clinical nursing audit; contributing to research; and supporting the primary and specialist nurses, the other two proposed levels of nurse working in the community. All of these functions have direct links with issues of accountability, and should incorporate a flexible response to local issues of health needs of clients/patients.

Record keeping

It is not uncommon to hear complaints about the amount of time spent by community nurses in writing up records and reports. However, record keeping is 'an essential and integral part of care and not a distraction from its provision' (UKCC 1993). In the community much of the interaction between professional and client/patient is unobserved, particularly in the home setting, so without good contemporaneous records accountability for care delivered is absent.

These records need to be meaningful. There is no place for the notoriously vague entry such as 'keeping well' or 'developing normally'. They should have accurate comprehensive entries particular to the client/patient at the time of contact. In the community the scope for understanding the impact of social and psychological factors on the individual is perhaps greater, and should be an integral part of the record. The danger of including such aspects is subjectivity of recording or reliance on information from another source – for instance another family member – without acknowledging that source. As many community nurses have realized, particularly health visitors in areas of child protection and safety, any such weakness or failure, for instance to record ineffectual visits, can lead to serious difficulties when professionals are required to give evidence in a court of law.

Accountability can be further developed through the use of records by demonstrating the purpose of the visit as well as the outcome and evaluation of whatever intervention took place. There is also a need to indicate future plans, so that future entries can indicate whether they were actually achieved. Most importantly, the element of partnership and the nature of the interaction with the client/patient should be documented so that their wishes and assessment are seen to be involved in the decision-making process.

Another development, building on the promotion of partnership between client and professional, that is happening in a piecemeal way throughout the country is client-held records. The impetus for this comes from a variety of sources including, in 1990, the implementation of the Act allowing access to health records. The Children's Act (1989) in England and Wales also emphasizes the ethos of sharing of information and enabling parents to become more equal partners with professionals in the care of their children. The Expert Maternity Group's recent report (1993) suggested that one of the indicators of success of maternity care adapting itself to the needs of women using the service would be that within 5 years all women should be entitled to carry their own notes. A natural progression of this would be enabling the women to hold the records of their children. The first principle for good maternity care noted in the report is recognizing the central role that the women should have in planning care for themselves and their babies, a philosophy which could certainly underpin and be translated to other areas of community nursing. Clearly, the professional is demonstrably more accountable to the client with open-access records: more open and honest relationships are facilitated and the progression to client-held records can only enhance this.

Within current writing 'audit', which is defined in *Chambers 20th Century Dictionary* as 'a calling to account', is another issue under discussion. Auditing of records offers the opportunity to debate, within peer groups, the individual service given against locally agreed standards of care. Given that many practitioners in the community are working in an isolated way, this is an ideal means of offering peer support and is useful in developing professional expertise. In areas where this approach has been tried, initial fears that it would result in criticism of personal practice have generally been unfounded, and instead it has provided a useful way of sharing and developing good practice.

Record keeping is also the means by which the individual practitioner offers a personal account to their manager and thus to the employing authority. This type of record keeping is very different from that described above and is an inadequate measure of care given, as it is largely a measurement of the quantity of work undertaken and not the quality. However, if used in conjunction with caseload and community/practice profiles, it can also help establish the level of service requirement.

CASE STUDY AND DISCUSSION

There is a tension between how accountability is seen by managers and how it is seen by professionals, the latter including both nurses who work in community settings and other members of the primary health-care team. Managers tend to view accountability in terms of 'externally imposed control', whereas professionals see it as a personal matter which derives from 'internalized professionalism' (Green 1992). Issues of professional autonomy pervade any discussion about accountability, such autonomy being seen by some to be threatened both by managerialism and by the 'enlightened consumer' who challenges the 'expert' (Williams *et al.* 1993)

Managerial accountability may be clearly linked to national and local targets for health care, which have recently been related to increasing the say of local communities in NHS decision making. Community profiling, already being undertaken by many community nurses, as mentioned previously, could certainly make a considerable contribution to setting such targets.

Taylor (1991) suggests that the development of smaller local units for service planning and provision, which are obliged to produce annual audits for the consumers and to have 'strong representation from the main user groups' would enhance the provision of sensitive care and offer 'real accountability to the community'.

Participation in care

The whole area of patient participation in care is one which has long been familiar to nurses who work in the community, not least because of the complete impossibility of *not* taking the wishes of individuals and their families into consideration when seeking to provide care to people in their own homes.

Community nurses work very much at the interface between the public and lay carers on the one hand, and management and other professionals on the other, and this creates particular dilemmas with regard to accountability. Health visiting in particular has striven for many years to clarify its remit as a profession that seeks to bridge the gap between professionals and recipients of care, consistently claiming an advocacy role and aiming to use health visiting expertise to represent and to empower clients. This is not a straightforward task; the following case study illustrates the complexity of accountability for nurses working in community settings and provides a helpful focus for subsequent discussion about teamwork and partnerships.

Case study

Mary is a 24-year-old single woman who was diagnosed about 2 years ago as having a compulsive–obsessional disorder. She is currently on antidepressants, which have helped her mood swings but not the obsessional symptoms, such as constant hairbrushing and bedmaking. She lives with her parents, has a baby (Megan) aged 5 months, and has had no contact with the child's father since she became aware that she was pregnant. The child is physically healthy and achieving the appropriate developmental milestones to date. Mary's mother (Jane) is heavily involved in Megan's care, and is contemplating giving up a part-time job in order to provide this care. Mary is keen to perform the role of mother, but is in some danger of being displaced by Jane, who is more confident and competent than Mary at present. A community psychiatric nurse was involved with the family in the antenatal period, but has since withdrawn and is now available for consultation if required. The role of the consultant psychiatrist has been primarily in diagnosis and treatment; he is also now on the periphery and will see Mary for review on a 3-monthly basis, unless the GP seeks advice or intervention at an earlier date.

This client lives on an isolated local authority housing estate which was built in the 1960s. There are no supportive resources in the area apart from a children's centre, run by the local social services department. The primary health-care team is based in a purpose-built health centre about a mile away from the client's home, and the general practitioners are non-fundholders. The consultant psychiatrist involved in the case is based in the local psychiatric hospital and the home help is based at the area social work department. A health visitor's management structure is outwith the health centre, and they are answerable to a clinical nurse manager who manages a number of community nurses working in this locality. It is fairly typical of care in the community that the various professionals involved are working alongside one another but within different management structures, which partially explains why professional autonomy is such a key issue for community practitioners.

In this case study the health visitor may be said to be accountable in various ways, from external factors such as networking abilities, knowledge of available resources and relationships with other members of the team, to a personal day-to-day relationship with the family.

Partnerships

It is useful to view the fulfilment of accountability in terms of participation and partnerships. There are three main partnerships evident here:

- partnership with the community, including its appropriate resources/services;
- partnership with others involved in supporting and caring for Mary and her child – including her mother Jane, who is very much at the centre of the web of support;
- partnership with Mary herself.

The cooperation of the other members of the multidisciplinary team depends, to a considerable extent, upon a shared understanding of the special contributions each person can make to the care of this family, as well as upon good communication skills. Such awareness and ability are required if a health visitor is to perform adequately in this situation, and require considerable skill and prior learning on their part.

Case discussions are essential to maximize helpful communication between members of the caring team and, in order to increase the clients' control over the situation, they should participate fully in such case discussions to assess the situation and plan for the future. Health visitors should also liaise with the home care supervisor as necessary, and the potential use of a children's centre placement would be on the basis of enabling Mary to develop her parenting skills.

Regular contact between the GP and the health visitor would enable them to share important information, preferably with the client's prior knowledge. One of the issues that frequently arises when working within a team is the day-to-day problem of deciding what information ought to be shared and with whom, given that the trust and confidence of a client is so important. For example, although the health visitor would also liaise with the home care supervisor in this particular case, they would not share the same type of information as would be shared with the general practitioner. This selective sharing of information should always be negotiated with the client. The possible use of a children's centre placement, in order to enable Mary to further develop her parenting skills, would also depend on considerable discussion and negotiation with Mary herself.

The relationship between the family and the health visitor is of central importance to the provision of sensitive and appropriate care – without a positive and helpful relationship there would be no way forward. This relationship will be successful only if it is flexible and dynamic, with the health visitor constantly seeking to share power and responsibility with her clients. Since her parents are such an important part of Mary's immediate environment, a major challenge for the health visitor is to build on the strengths of the family, encouraging Jane to withdraw gradually from directly caring for her grandchild but remaining involved in an appropriate way and consistently fostering Mary's confidence in her ability to care for her own child. In this particular team of carers the health visitor probably has the greatest opportunity to develop a constructive long-term relationship, which will enhance the wellbeing of the whole family. District nurses share this privileged position of long-term involvement with many of their clients, allowing a gradual aggregation of knowledge about how the families in their caseload function. Unfortunately, there is little research evidence to explain how community nurses gather and utilize knowledge for the benefit of their clients (Lightfoot *et al.* 1992)

It is essential that the health visitor involved in this case keeps clear records which include events, case discussions and observations of relationships, especially between Megan and her mother. The health visitor's own role should be documented, evaluating interventions and the expected purpose of future contacts. Such records would also serve to monitor the progress of Megan's growth and development, as well as indicating either Mary's growing self-confidence and parenting skills or her need for enhanced support.

Developing a useful working partnership with Mary is at the heart of this case study, a task which will require knowledge, expertise, commitment and the direct involvement of the health visitor. Clauses 9.5 and 9.6 of the UKCC code (1992a), regarding inappropriate delegation to others which compromises the interests of the client, are pertinent. For example, if skill mix was being promoted in this locality, how could a less skilled nurse usefully contribute in a case such as this? In some districts, nursery nurses with additional training that enables them to work with families in the community, have been used to offer additional support and foster parenting skills (Marks 1993). Projects such as these have demonstrated that the judicial use of other skilled staff has proved to be useful in community nurse teams.

CONCLUSION

Working in the community brings with it greater opportunities for professional autonomy and freedom. The satisfaction of building long-term relationships with clients and becoming familiar with the character of a community and understanding its impact upon clients and their families is integral to the nature of daily practice. The current focus on community care and nursing, with all the changes in progress and those that are envisaged, creates chances for reviewing and developing enhanced practice as well as the consequent uncertainty that change brings. It is easy for professionals living through organizational changes in service and practice to become inward looking and concerned for their own working conditions. While acknowledging these difficulties, the focus must remain upon clients and their families, with the issues of accountability in all its various guises remaining at the core of daily practice.

Working with children: accountability and paediatric nursing

9

Gosia Brykczynska

INTRODUCTION

Nurses are constantly being told that they are responsible and, above all, accountable for their professional practice. It is less clear, however, what is meant by the words 'responsible' or 'accountable'. Styles (1985), in an interesting article on the nature of accountability, rightly points out that 'as a word gains popularity it loses clarity. Accountability is one such endangered word'. Not only is the word concept not clearly understood by those who would appear to be most obviously affected by it but, depending on the professional and/or vocational outlook of the user of the word, it may take on quite varying and specific connotations. Thus, for modern health-care workers 'accountability' has about it an inevitable ring of testimony and reporting – a rather defensive reaction to some past event; a reporting back of junior to senior professional. Philosophers, however, see accountability mainly through the prism of its chief constituent or, as Bergman (1981) noted, its 'key component', that is, responsibility.

This chapter gives an analysis of accountability in relationship to paediatric nursing and child care, presenting first some definitions of paediatric nursing and then of children, in order to set the context for a review of accountability based on Bergman's (1981) schema for nursing accountability.

Bergman (1981), in analysing the dimensions of accountability, saw the need for a necessary hierarchical infrastructure to be in place in order for true professional accountability to be possible. Thus, what Bergman (1981) refers to as ability, that is, skills and values, philosophers refer to rather globally as know-ledge, particularly personal knowledge – or as Russell (1991) said, 'knowledge by acquaintance'. Most health-care professionals tend to talk of the necessity for 'authority' to act, that is, authority which is vested in the moral agent by virtue of their rank, education, charisma or legal power. To have authority therefore implies freedom to act in particular and specific autonomous ways as required, and freedom justifiably to be able, at one's request, to expect certain acts to be performed. There is no real authority unless one has freedom to manoeuvre, freedom to choose certain acts, and freedom to go down certain paths (Glover 1970; Nuttall 1993).

It is only when ability and authority are adequately matched that one can start analysing the true nature of responsibility, which in turn contributes to the profession's understanding of accountability for practice. This schema of Bergman's (1981) will be presented within the context of paediatric nursing concerns.

Definition of paediatric nursing

Paediatric nurses have a wide remit. Not only do they accommodate sick chil-dren, but also take under their wing healthy children and work with them and their families in order to maintain their health, in schools, clinics and outpatient departments; in fact, they are concerned with the health and wellbeing of the whole child, wherever it may be (Glasper and Tucker 1993). Traditionally, paediatric nursing has been the branch of nursing which, by convention, has as its focus of concern the ill or potentially ill child. As such, paediatric nurses focused on the ill child, from neonates to adolescents. More recently, however, as a better understanding of the nature of childhood has emerged, with a clearer understanding of disease aetiology, paediatric nurses are expanding their sphere of concerns.

Newly educated paediatric nurses following the Project 2000 educational programme will be qualified 'all-round' generically educated child-health nurses, with a new scope of practice that necessitates a re-evaluation of the traditional terms of paediatric nursing accountability (Fradd 1990). Paediatric nursing is a special branch of professional nursing requiring specific knowledge and skills, within which one can specialize even further, for example in paedi-atric oncology nursing, community nursing, school nursing or intensive care.

Although it may appear uncomplicated to describe the extent and scope of paediatric nursing, it is somewhat more complex to adequately describe its client group. Notions of childhood, according to some historians, are relatively recent, and indeed in some parts of the world an individual over the age of 6 or 7 is accorded a place in society akin to that reserved for adults elsewhere (Archard 1993; James and Prout 1990). Children are considered to be smaller versions of adults, and have to compete with them for natural resources and contribute very early in their life to the economic wellbeing of their society. In such societies there rarely exists the notion of adolescence as we know it. In contemporary European and industrial settings, the demands on the nurse working with children and their families help to shape and orient the nurse's understanding of professional accountability. Unlike those working with otherwise sentient adults, the paediatric nurse (together with all those health workers engaged in caring for members of vulnerable groups) must always bear in mind the cooperative and, in some cases, coopted caring role alongside that of parents and legally defined primary carers.

Accountability in this context is not just moral responsibility for personal, or even collective, action. It must also always be for facilitating and empowering families and the children themselves to be accountable and ready to share in the responsibilities of health maintenance, promotion and restoration. Precisely because children are not held fully responsible for their actions, professional adults who come into contact with children must start to initiate them into increasing their levels of responsibility for their actions and decisions.

Accountability for health-care decisions in a paediatric context, if it is to be patient centred, must always be a form of shared collective responsibility between various professional groups, the family, the child and society, where the latter outlines the framework within which accountability can and must be discussed.

ABILITY

It seems obvious that, in order to be held accountable for actions and decisions, one needs to be capable of discerning correct acts and decisions and be prepared (skilled and schooled) to do so. It is interesting that many contemporary philosophers discuss (if only to proceed further) the reasoning that lay behind Aristotle's strong condemnation of those individuals who make incorrect choices, even if these were made under duress (Aristotle 1962; Lloyd 1969). Aristotle differentiated between the universal moral knowledge that one ought to have (and should be striving to continually expand and cultivate), and specific knowledge, which might legitimately be missing. The general universal knowledge (of right and wrong) is so fundamental to the nature of the mature moral agent that there is little one can say by way of excuse to mitigate a wrong choice or act. Likewise, in paediatric nursing certain knowledge is considered 'universal': all qualified paediatric nurses must know the difference between a normal neonatal heart rate and a toddler's, or levels of expected social development in an 8-year-old and an adolescent. What would be specific knowledge for an 'outsider' is considered not only routine and basic in paediatrics but, in fact, part of the accepted universal backdrop against which decisions can and should be made, and against which the paediatric nurse can be held accountable. Should a paediatric nurse not know (i.e. did not have that level of competence and ability), by that same deficiency they would be declaring themselves outside the fraternity of professional paediatric nursing. In order to be held professionally accountable one must therefore have at least a minimum level of competency and skill relevant to that profession or discipline.

Aristotle, referring to Greek citizens, expected of them a basic universal level of moral discernment in order for them to be held morally responsible. In the same way, in the example of specialized professional practice there is a universal body of knowledge that one must possess in order to practise one's art. This knowledge carries with it certain obligations.

Obligations

One of the many obligations or responsibilities that go with the knowledge of a child's psychosocial development may be that of a certain measure of political activism, in order to ensure that children in society receive their minimum rights. This type of social and professional awareness may mean lobbying local councils or health authorities for better facilities for children. Alternatively, it may mean closer liaison with other child-care workers, e.g. play-leaders, nursery school teachers etc. to acquire greater access for underprivileged children to childminding facilities. Certainly, knowledge of the needs of children does not finish at the end of an 8-hour shift in a local district hospital. Basic 'universal' paediatric knowledge will permeate one's whole approach. It forms part of one's value system and, therefore, is fundamental to child welfare and the ethical decision-making process.

Accountability in a paediatric context is for consistent concern about the welfare of children. Such a high level of knowledge and commitment, however, does not come vicariously. It falls upon professional paediatric nurse lecturers to inculcate, not only the requisite level of paediatric values that form the moral core of paediatric nursing, but also the necessary amount of paediatric science and care to its students. As Cook (1990) observed, 'If nursing education is the core of the profession, the nurse educationalists have a responsibility to the practitioner, the helper and the manager, since they must, to some extent, provide the knowledge and skills for the professionals to become accountable'. That nurses need a certain level of competency in order to be held accountable for creative, positive practice seems reasonable, but what about the parents who share in the child's care?

Involving parents

Modern paediatric nursing is practised together with a child's parents, and accountability for paediatric practice includes a concept of collective accountability of all those working with a child – not only qualified professionals. The most important beings in the life of a child are the parents, and they will also bear the greatest share of moral responsibility for that child. The relevant question to ask must be: what level of expertise and ability can be expected of parents in order for them to be considered 'accountable', with the nurse, for the care of a child?

The educative role of nursing is well documented and, starting with educative antenatal classes, prospective parents are helped and guided, as necessary, by nursing professionals right through the period of their child's infancy and childhood. Parents, however, may quickly outstrip professionals in specific knowledge of their child. This is certainly the case as regards habits, social customs, preferences and even where physiological norms are concerned. The educative role of the professional in such circumstances is, literally, to fill in the gaps, in order for the parents to make a coherent picture that will enable them to continue caring for and being responsible for their own child. It is all the more interesting, therefore, that many professionals in the health-care field still regard parents' knowledge and abilities with considerable suspicion: even, on occasion, with derision. Alderson (1990), in her landmark book *Choosing for Children*, about parental informed consent for children, documents well the attitude of some surgeons to the decision-making capacities of parents. Thus she records one consultant as saying:

'Don't expect much of parents. Some are good witnesses and some are vague and not terribly helpful. In episodic events I may rely on them, but I tell them what is likely to happen, that the child may become blue...It's a way of handling it and involving parents. I don't rely on their opinion. I prefer to go on objective clinical data' (Alderson 1990).

Obviously the surgeon is clinically responsible for performing the right operation at the right time, but it is the parents who have to agree to the surgery and are accountable in society for caring for their child and providing adequate medical care. The level of parental accountability for making correct decisions, and appropriately caring for their child, is immeasurably increased and augmented by the intervention and cooperation, if not the advocacy, of paediatric nurses.

This truism is most clearly demonstrated when it is absent. The parent who refuses reasonable treatment for a child is an obvious example. Even more startling are the instances where, unfortunately, nurses agree with parents about decisions not to treat a child for an otherwise treatable disorder or symptom (even if the proposed treatment is only palliative). Accountability of parents for their children's welfare is paramount – and it is considered in law to be a responsibility rather than a right. This observation was upheld by the High Court in the Gillick case, where Lord Scarman told Mrs Gillick that, in effect, she only had parental rights over her children as long as she also fulfilled her parental responsibilities (i.e. those of parenting) and was actively involved in parenting her children (Dyer 1985). The fundamental task of paediatric nurses is to work with parents so that they can continue parenting their child throughout its illness and childhood, and be in a reasonable position to be accountable for the care given to their child. In many respects modern paediatric nursing is care delivered by proxy; accountability is, therefore, also referred out to parents, to the extent that they have been given the necessary skills and competence to do so by paediatric nurses (Alderson 1990; Fradd 1990).

Autonomy of children

If paediatric nurses share with parents the accountability for a young patient's welfare, what personal decision-making skills and aptitudes are required for the child to be considered an autonomous, competent moral agent? Certainly some children, as some adults, can be held accountable for cooperation with the health-care team (Alderson 1993). Thus, even fairly young children with spina bifida can be taught how to self-catheterize and look after their basic needs and report to the school nurse as and when appropriate. It is no longer the responsibility of the parent or the nurse to ensure continence once the child has learnt the requisite skills and is deemed competent to function independently at school. The child takes over responsibility for that area of their life. Good nursing accountability, however, demands that the child knows it has access to a school nurse, and that the nurse is aware of the child's progress and is concerned with liaising between the child, its parents, its school and the referral centre.

Children who have long-term illnesses, for example diabetes or asthma, can be held accountable for self-medication and, in cooperation with the school nurse, take on essentially adult health-care responsibilities as and when appropriate. A nurse, or a member of the community child health team, in such an instance is held accountable for ensuring that such children and their parents are given the necessary guidance; that there is access to emergency care; and that relevant adults, such as teachers, know how to intervene appropriately, and so on. In all these cases the child is slowly introduced to the world of adult responsibilities as far as their health-care needs are concerned, for such an approach truly respects the child as an individual who is capable (when appropriately prepared) to take on such responsibilities in respect to their competencies (Alderson 1993).

There is a natural tendency to shield the ill person from a bad prognosis, an uncertain diagnosis, or simply from partaking in decision-making. Sometimes even active cooperation with a treatment protocol by the patient is frowned upon. The patient is expected to be entirely passive. There is, however, an essential paradox here, for in order to really cooperate adequately with a treatment – that is, to make a positive difference to health – one needs to be involved in treatment plans, be aware of one's diagnosis and agree to protocols. Few examples of the potential burden of this duty are more poignant than when telling a patient that they are not likely to survive an illness. In the context of paediatric nursing the question arises as to who takes on this responsibility, and to what extent a child should know that they are dying. Can one actually be ethically accountable for imparting such information to a child? Children, as much as adults, like to be in control of their lives and their own affairs. To the extent that they are capable of this they are likewise accountable to their family and society for their brief lives.

As one mother recounts, she imparted to her adolescent son Hamish the information about his impending death with a certain amount of trepidation, albeit with far more authority and love than any professional paediatric worker ever could. Thus she recounts:

'Two or so days before he died, I manoeuvred separate conversations with both our children that imparted that knowledge to them. Hamish reacted not with fear or horror, but as if he had just been told he should go for a walk on a very stormy day – 'Mama, I'd really rather not' (Cooper and Harpin 1991).

Responsibility for imparting important information to children should normally lie with the parents, who will obviously need a lot of support and help from professionals. In keeping with the entire ethos of modern child-centred paediatric care, it is hard to envisage treating a child who does not know his or her diagnosis (Alderson 1990, 1993). Paediatric nurses' accountability lies in supporting the parents in this role – and only when the parents cannot perform this task should they step in (Casey 1993). Assessment of the parents' competence to take over this hitherto traditionally professional task lies within the remit of good paediatric nursing and medicine.

AUTHORITY

It has often been said that there can be no accountability for practice where there is no true autonomy of action. If actions are performed under undue duress, or tasks omitted because of lack of choice, then moral philosophers would start to question the level of freedom and free will a person is experiencing. We can only be accountable for that over which we as individuals exercise a degree of authority (Glover 1970; French 1993; Nuttall 1993).

Authority, in the context of paediatric nursing, can be either the nurses' personal authority over their own actions, stemming at least in part from expertise and in part from invested hierarchical structures; or authority that a nurse vests in the parents, who are the child's main caregivers. Thus, as with competence, it is not only the nurse's authority that is being discussed but also the patient's and their family's. The nurse, in truth, has no authority to act for or with a child except that granted to her by the parents and, increasingly, by the child (Alderson 1993; HM Government 1989, 1991; Tingle 1990c, 1991). This shift in the focus of authority, and therefore in moral perspective, is extremely important, for it is not the nurses' authority and level of free will over their own actions that is solely at stake, but the level of autonomy and authority the young patient and their family have over their actions that are of paramount importance in paediatric nursing (Alderson 1993).

Free will and choice

Issues of free will are central to arguments pertaining to moral behaviour, for without sufficient free will there can be no discussion about moral choices. If mature individuals are to be responsible for their actions they must be able to choose those behaviours and to act in those ways that support their moral intentions (Glover 1970; Nuttall 1993). Nurses often say that they would like to behave in a certain way, to conduct themselves in a particular fashion, but do not have the freedom or authority to do so. It is difficult to talk of accountability for practice if there is no corresponding authority of action to match the level of competency and insight (Lanara 1982).

Aristotle, in his *Nicomachean Ethics*, was not particularly lenient with people who stated that they behaved against their better judgement under duress. He felt that it was important to structure one's life in such a way as to be more in control more of the time and that unpleasantness may have to be a consequence of making an ethical decision, that is, some morally correct judgements may be unpleasant. Often we complain about lack of authority to act in the way we would like to, when in reality we have not done all that we could to structure our environment to be more conducive to a particular ethical milieu (Aristotle 1962; Lanara 1982).

Power and political action

Perhaps one of the most stressful situations in nursing is having the knowledge and skills to direct specific action, but to feel deprived of the power to influence and promote necessary change (Lanara 1982; Styles 1985; Fradd 1990). Paediatric nurses have long known that small children need to be nursed in purpose-designed paediatric specialty wards. Children fare better when looked after by their parents on wards catering to their specific needs. In spite of this accepted child-centred wisdom, there is no legal power to back up its implications (ASC 1987; Central Health Services Council 1991).

If a hospital or community trust does not want to provide separate accident and emergency services, or separate ear, nose and throat specialty beds serviced by paediatric nurses, then paediatric nurses themselves do not have the power to create change. Such situations, where personal knowledge of professionally correct conduct clashes with management realities, highlights the essential impotence that nurses feel. Paediatric nurses, however, are not altogether without influence and, together with parent interest groups, can and should lobby for particular changes.

Ultimately, power and authority comes to those who actively seek it. Consumer groups, such as ASC, formerly National Association for the Welfare of Children in Hospital (NAWCH), have developed, over the past 25 years, an authority base which few modern governments would dare to totally ignore. Lobby groups may not have the last say, but in a democratic society they do represent the vested power of an otherwise voiceless group. Action for Sick Children, together with the Paediatric Society of the Royal College of Nursing and the British Paediatricians Association (BPA), have co-written several significant consultation and advisory documents laying out the philosophy and orientation of modern child-centred health care.

Eventually, governments will have to accommodate the recommendations of these groups. The authority of modern paediatric nurses is not necessarily self-generated: rather, it stems from a concerted effort to be in tandem with parental thinking, other child-centred groups and, obviously, children themselves. The old adage that there is power (and authority) in numbers has much to recommend it. The central problem with all child-care services is that children form roughly a quarter of the entire population and yet take up a very small percentage of the health-care budget.

It is a constant political temptation to marginalize paediatric services and reduce the paediatric health-care budget because, the argument goes, at the end of the day children cannot speak up for themselves and do not have the power to vote. Authority and power to influence child health-centred change comes, paradoxically, not from interested third parties – that is, paediatric health-care workers – but from children and parents themselves, who are seriously taking on board accountability for their own health-care needs. As long as authority to act was seen solely as the province of health-care workers, the possible variations in the delivery of health care were predictable.

Now that children themselves and their parents are demanding a greater share in the say about health-care structures, and are voicing their own authoritative demands, it is impossible to foretell all the consequences of this approach. Shared collective responsibility should itself lower overall anxieties and concerns related to paediatric health-care provision. This is a creative collective response to the moral imperative to care, in partnership with the parents of sick children (Fradd 1990; Casey 1993; Alderson 1990, 1993).

RESPONSIBILITY

Much has been written about the importance of responsibility in connection with accountability. Nurses are encouraged to be responsible for their nursing actions, as conscious responsibility will contribute to overall higher levels of accountability. It is interesting that Lanara (1982) defines responsibility as being 'dependent upon knowledge, discretion, judgement, and the ability to make decisions about one's work'. She sees responsibility as something over which the informed, reflective nurse has considerable control. Philosophers, however, are not so uniformly sure about levels and the nature of responsibility.

To be responsible implies being answerable, or accountable, to either another or oneself for some act or acts. Responsibility implies moral accountability for one's actions, a capability for rational conduct, and for fulfilling obligations for vested trust; it means justifying a trust; to be reliable. Such dictionary definitions, however, obscure some of the more complex questions associated with the proposition.

As the philosopher Peter French (1993) comments, for many people 'a person is morally responsible for what he has done only if he could have done otherwise', a proposition not altogether foreign to the average moral agent working in a health-care context. This sentiment presupposes two fundamental premises in the discourse concerning responsibility, namely, that the moral agent is acting in good faith with free will – that is, uncoerced; and secondly, that there is a known (or even unknown) choice available. There is an emphasis in this particular presentation of responsibility on free will and choice, two moral ingredients which are not necessarily always present or in fact capable of being equally present.

French (1993) calls this situation the principle of alternative possibilities (PAP), but PAP most evidently cannot always be honoured. Many professionally morally correct acts, resulting from a measure of responsibility, are undertaken in the knowledge of either no acceptable alternatives or, indeed, any other alternative, given a desired objective.

Responsibility and treatment

Thus, to treat a child for common lymphocytic leukaemia will involve discomfort, and no known protocol exists that will change this fact. Moral responsibility for treating a leukaemic child with minimum side-effects requires not so much choices from among protocol treatments, as the courage to treat the child via a painful process in the face of a growing emphasis on the sole reliance on alternative folk medicines.

Several years ago a health visitor, against universally accepted wisdom, encouraged a mother to discontinue taking her child to the oncology clinic. The nurse was rightly held morally responsible for contributing to the untimely death of the child, if not being an agent of manslaughter. She was held responsible even though she claimed she was working with the mother, and had felt she had no other choice she could have made. The same could be said of a Jehovah's Witness parent whose child requires a blood transfusion. The fact that the parent's religion curtails the range of medical interventions they may feel comfortable about adopting does not absolve them from moral responsibility for refusing treatment that requires blood transfusions. It is, perhaps, good to repeat the often-quoted truism that in a moral context to do nothing is to choose to do something, and that 'something is a morally and legally binding choice' (Tingle 1990c, 1991).

Liability and responsibility

Responsibility can also be seen as a form of liability. For some people, responsibility is a bothersome addition to morality which can curb overzealous righteousness, or it may prompt action where otherwise they would be passive. It can also be likened to a barter game, as French (1993) proposes, since 'we spend a considerable (perhaps inordinate) amount of time trying to avoid responsibility wherever and whenever possible'. The need to avoid responsibility and the act of passing it to someone else stem from the logical deduction that responsibility involves accepting obligations and performing actions for which one can be held accountable. As French (1993) astutely observes: 'no wonder that avoidance of responsibility has become almost an art form, one that is learned and practised relatively early in life and honed to the end'.

It is quite natural to strive to avoid responsibility, even if increased responsibility means considerably more kudos and economic remuneration. Paediatric nurses, traditionally, have not gone out of their way to court responsibility, but much is changing. With a new emphasis on the need for increased skills and hands-on therapeutic interventions, paediatric nurses are realizing that there may be a correspondingly greater level of responsibility but also, more specifically, a perceptually increased level of work satisfaction. As French (1993) noted: 'People merit praise and blame for what they do, and not just 'on the basis' of what they do'.

Consequences of responsibility

Translated into nursing language, paediatric nurses are found to be accountable and are deemed responsible, with corresponding praise or blame, in direct proportion as they are seen to behave in praiseworthy or blameful fashion. It is not the profession of paediatric nursing, however, that is under scrutiny but the specific conduct of particular nurses. French (1993) claims that 'the responsibility barter game (RBG) is probably the most common experience ordinary people have with morality', since it is the aim of everyone, including nurses, to avoid and pass on all possible extraneous responsibility, in spite of any possible benefits (and there usually are some) that might ensue from increased obligations and accountability.

Few people are as aware of the ramifications of increased responsibilities as health-care workers and paediatric nurses. They are also aware of the increased prestige and gratification that accompany increased (extended) role performance. Nonetheless, although it would seem that increased responsibility should be everyone's aim and ambition, it is a factor for individual negotiation rather than a foregone conclusion based on a decree from superior managers. As French (1993) observes, 'Peoples lives are affected when responsibility is ascribed, assessed and accepted'; it has profound moral implications for the actors in the game and, on balance, the less direct responsibility and the more indirect credit one has, the better one feels. No-one wants to manage an under-staffed paediatric intensive care unit, but nurses readily bask in the public praise heaped on 'heroic angels' fighting to save babies' lives.

Curiously, as French (1993) notes, too much praise is also to be avoided, perhaps because of the fickle nature of public opinion, and it is altogether seen to be more psychologically stable to avoid as much positive as negative public-ity and comment. There is, of course, another, much more deep-seated reason why praise and blame for accepted responsibility are felt to be uncomfortable: it is very difficult to be sure of the true motives behind someone's actions and, therefore, for an action for which we are responsible by virtue of our profession to be seen as praiseworthy and/or exceptional. The motive behind the action would need to be something above and beyond the call of duty and akin to a type of heroism.

Few paediatric nurses can claim to work entirely from altruistic motives. Motives for moral actions are usually mixed and demonstrate, in the same person at any one time, varying degrees of moral and personal interest. How often do nurses dismiss praise (even routine praise) with the disclaimer 'Oh, that was nothing, was doing my duty...' or, 'That was nothing, anyone would have done likewise', even though they represent in their persons many years of professional training. They have often put much of themselves into the task at hand, and in truth, not everyone would have done what had just been performed! It is, therefore, not just a matter of false humility as French (1993) observed: it also has something to do with this deep-seated desire to hold on to as little responsibility as possible; after all, this time it paid off, but next time might be different!

It is not just paediatric nurses who have to grapple with responsibility and accountability: parents and children are also inextricably linked in the responsi-bility barter game. Just as nurses are finding that they are responsible for ever-increasing and invading professional work, so too parents and children are cajoled, and even encouraged, to take on ever more responsibility for their participation in health matters with health-care workers (Fradd 1990; Alderson 1993; Casey 1993).

Responsibility of parents and children

Parents and children are asked to take on ever more responsibility without necessarily more obvious benefits or rights, except that it would appear that parents desire to continue with their parenting responsibilities and looking after their children, even in hospital (Casey 1993). Parents see this not only as an ongoing burden but also as a parental right. Child health, in this context, becomes a shared responsibility between various professional and non-profes-sional adults.

The child, too, has a measure of responsibility. Children traditionally have been denied responsibility on the premise that they are not capable of being fully responsible and, therefore, accountable for their acts. According to French (1993), in order to qualify as a player of the responsibility barter game the player must be a member of the moral community, which implies a particular level of moral and social development. Presumably, players once 'in the game' can be voted out, or temporarily disqualify themselves by virtue of disease, unconsciousness or lack of sobriety.

Children, additionally, have to prove that they possess relevant moral and social knowledge. One cannot hold children accountable for the maintenance of their own good dental health unless and until they are capable of understanding the significance and have the requisite skills of daily dental hygiene and adequate nutrition.

One related question that troubles child sociologists, psychologists and moral philosophers concerns the nature of the loss of innocence (Archard 1993; James and Prout 1990). Rephrased, the argument suggests that we should be concerned that the price of being held responsible for our actions means an automatic loss of 'innocence'. Conversely, some would say that what a child does not know about harmful bacteria, for example, does not concern it, at least not directly. Personal knowledge brings with it personal responsibility and a loss of innocence. French (1993), however, points out that losing innocence is connected with gaining maturity and moral development, and that moral innocence is more akin to moral 'virginity' than moral purity. As he rightly points out, innocence is a matter of moral status, the status of someone not mature enough to be a fully 'paid-up' member of the moral community. It is not a condition that adults need, or indeed should yearn for, even though as he notes 'innocence...is only valued by those who no longer possess it' (French 1993).

Innocence absolves from responsibility, but only temporarily, as it is the duty and responsibility of adults who are collectively responsible before society, to instil in children the universal concepts of right and wrong and the nature of good and evil. Once 'moral innocence' is lost there is no going back: paradise can never be regained. Loss of moral 'virginity' is irrecoverable, since knowledge about oneself can only, by definition, be an active ongoing process (French 1993). Thus, an asthmatic child taught by parents and the community paediatric nurse to use an inhaler, cannot go back on its knowledge and behave as if it never knew what to do in the event of an asthmatic attack. Most children guard their autonomy and newly learnt skills, and do not see them as a loss of innocence so much as a necessary growth and move in the direction of maturity and self-determination. For this reason, many children who are taught how to use an inhaler, or to administer their own insulin, will not take kindly to giving up this responsibility to a teacher or camp director when the class goes on an outing or a camping trip. With this responsibility comes the right to real – albeit limited – self-determination. It is difficult to argue with a child who has already been given responsibility as to why this responsibility should necessarily change and/or stop (Alderson 1993).

Responsibility can therefore be seen as the most crucial element in the accountability equation, and one shared in proportion to moral development by children as well as adults. Thus, paediatric nurses in the course of their work are not only responsible for their own actions but also for the upholding of parents' ongoing responsibilities and the development of a child's own sense of responsibility. Accountability, for paediatric nurses, rests on a delicate balance of their professional responsibilities with those of parents and children, where the child's 'responsibilities' and self-determination will always be paramount, as it is the child who is at the centre of every paediatric nurse's concerns.

CONCLUSION

As the poet Emily Dickinson warns us, we are to combine authority and power with our professional knowledge. This is the case if we are not to renege on our responsibilities for child-centred paediatric nursing practice. Just as:

'A bone has obligations,
A being has the same
A marrowless assembly
Is culpabler than shame' (Emily Dickinson 1957).

Paediatric nurses must therefore put courage and conviction behind their shared co-accountability with parents and children for increased child health.

PART FOUR:

Legal and Ethical Issues

The legal accountability of the nurse

10

John H. Tingle

INTRODUCTION

The broad aim of this chapter is to analyse the legal accountability of the nurse. There will be a discussion of the nature of law and the meaning of accountability within the context of practical nursing situations, and in order to illustrate the wider effects of law in the NHS there will be a discussion of how the courts have responded to legal claims brought by patients and/or clients who have demanded an allocation of health-care resources or have alleged negligence because of their inadequate provision.

THE IMPORTANCE OF LEGAL ACCOUNTABILITY

The law affects everybody and it is something which cannot be ignored. Legal accountability is the prime form of accountability for every citizen, and nurses, like all other professionals, are personally accountable through the law for their actions or omissions. This individual legal accountability is channelled through the criminal and civil law and the courts.

The law maintains an important presumption: that ignorance of it will not excuse should legal action result. Therefore, as a matter of practical necessity nurses, like all other professionals, need to be aware of the legal aspects of their role. The nurse's legal accountability also needs to be contrasted with the other forms of accountability that exist – and these can conflict with each other. It is also possible to view some as being more important than others.

Interest, rights and duties: the role of the law

The law performs a number of general functions in society. It articulates interests, rights and duties and chooses between them when they conflict, and the case of Re S. (1992) provides a good illustration of this point. Sir Stephen Brown, President of the Family Division, granted a declaration that doctors could perform an emergency caesarean section on a woman aged 30 who urgently needed the operation to save her life and that of her unborn child, but who refused consent on religious grounds; the operation was performed against her wishes. Many interests can be seen to be at stake in this case: those of the mother, her other children and the unborn child. It could be said here that the law had protected the greatest number of interests.

Dispute resolution, compensation and punishment

The law is also used to resolve disputes, for example where a patient may have been injured by a nurse and sues for compensation. A practice nurse, for example, may have syringed an ear negligently (Parker and Wilson 1992) and caused the patient injury. The nurse may deny negligence, and if the case is not settled beforehand the dispute will be resolved in court.

Establishing nursing negligence

The important issues to be determined in the case stated above will be, first, whether the practice nurse owed a legal duty of care to the patient (Tingle 1990a). Broadly speaking, a legal duty of care is owed to our neighbours: people to whom we are proximate and who we can reasonably foresee will be injured by our actions or omissions. In the doctor–nurse–patient relationship this first element will nearly always be established. There is a sufficiently close, proximate relationship between nurse and patient to say that, generally speaking, a legal duty of care will always be owed.

Secondly, breach of the legal duty to care has to be established and the basic premise of the reasonable practice nurse would probably be used in the case in order to assess the appropriate legal standard of care to be exercised. The court would seek to find out whether the nurse acted as an ordinary skilled practice nurse would have acted in the circumstances of the case. Expert nurse evidence would be given on this point and the court might look for the exercise of a medical standard of care in the circumstances (Tingle 1993a). Regard would also be had as to the conduct of the delegating GP: in other words, whether there was any evidence of wrongful delegation (General Medical Council 1993). If unreasonable, negligent conduct is established, the person making the claim (the plaintiff) will then have to establish the third element, i.e. that the injuries received by the patient were caused, or materially contributed to by, the negligent conduct of the defendant or defendants. The harm must also have been reasonably foreseeable, and if all this is established and the court finds negligence then monetary compensation in the form of damages will be awarded.

Vicarious liability

The GP employer of the practice nurse will also be liable for the negligence, the appropriate term to use here being vicarious liability, which operates to make an employer liable, along with the employee, for any negligence caused by the employee. The negligent practice nurse, however, still remains personally legally liable for any wrongs and could still be sued personally by the injured patient.

The aim of the law

The aim of the law in personal injury court actions, where a breach of duty has been proved, is to try and compensate the physically injured plaintiff (the patient in the above example) as fully as money possibly can for the injuries received, i.e to put the plaintiff in the position they would have been in had the wrong not been committed (Tingle 1990b). It is very difficult to put into monetary terms the value of a lost sense or faculty, but nevertheless an attempt is made.

In criminal law the focus of the law is different because of the fundamental nature of what has occurred. The convicted person is seen as having committed a crime against society, and therefore society punishes. In civil law the defendant is viewed as having committed a wrong against an individual, therefore civil law is largely concerned with compensation, whereas criminal law is largely concerned with punishment.

Regulation, deterrence and education: the role of the law

The law has other general functions, such as deterrence, regulation and education.

The deterrent function

This operates when professionals see what happens to others who are negligent or commit crimes. They do not wish to be in the same unenviable position and will reflect on their professional practice and alter it if necessary.

The regulation function

This operates to check professional bodies like the UKCC (United Kingdom Central Council for Nursing, Midwifery and Health Visiting), Health Authorities, NHS trusts and other statutory organizations. For example, a health authority may be exercising its powers unlawfully and its actions could be challenged in a court and declared illegal.

The education function

This operates when court cases are reported in the professional nursing and legal literature, whereby more people become aware of the issues and will reflect on their professional practice and alter it if necessary. This education function can usefully be illustrated by the case of Crawford v. Board of Governors of Charing Cross Hospital, reported in *The Times* of 8 December 1953 (Tingle 1990b). The plaintiff, Mr Robert Joseph Crawford, was admitted to hospital for an operation to remove his bladder. The operation involved a blood transfusion and his arm was extended at an angle of 80° from his body so that he could be given the transfusion. He suffered a loss of power in his arm, was later found to be suffering from brachial palsy, and sued for negligence. The judge in the lower court based his finding of negligence on the anaesthetist's failure to read an article in *The Lancet* which warned of the danger of brachial palsy in these circumstances. The Court of Appeal allowed the appeal and found no negligence. Lord Denning stated that it would be putting too high a burden on a person to say that they must read every article in the medical press, although there could be a case of negligence where a recommendation becomes so well proven, accepted and known that it should have been read.

If a contributor makes a point in a journal it could be negligence to just rush in and adopt the findings, and much depends on how widely accepted and regarded the research or article is. Mason and McCall Smith (1994) analyse Crawford and its current implications:

'Failure to read a single article, it was said, may be excusable, while disregard of a series of warnings in the medical press could well be evidence of negligence. In view of the rapid progress currently being made in many areas of medicine, and in view of the amount of information confronting the average doctor, it is unreasonable to expect a doctor to be aware of every development in his field. At the same time, he must be reasonably up to date and must know of major developments.'

It is an essential element of the professional and legal accountability of nurses that they keep reasonably up to date in their field of professional nursing practice.

The law affects all aspects of nursing

The law affects all aspects of nursing practice, from making a cup of tea to giving injections. In the case of Pargeter v. Kensington and Chelsea and Westminster Health Authority, reported in *The Lancet* of 10 November 1979, a patient was given a cup of tea the day after having an operation to remove a cataract. He drank the tea, vomited immediately and his left eye burst open. Despite further corrective operations he eventually lost the sight in that eye. The patient sued for damages but was unsuccessful because negligence could not be established. A number of issues were discussed in the case, including the practice of testing the patient's tolerance to liquids by giving trial sips. The judge felt that in this case it was highly improbable that the common surgical nursing practice of giving trial sips of liquid had not been followed.

In the case of Smith v. Brighton and Lewes Hospital Management Committee, reported in *The Times Law Report* of 1 May 1958, the plaintiff received injuries when a course of streptomycin injections overran. The nursing sister was found to be negligent in not taking elementary precautions to stop this, and damages were awarded. She could have drawn a red line or a star on the treatment sheet to indicate the time when the prescription was to end. Since she did not do this, extra doses were accidentally given by two other nurses.

A number of the functions of law have been identified and discussed and related to aspects of nursing practice. This process will be continued later in the chapter, when the nurse's role in health-care resource allocation is discussed along with how the courts have become involved in these issues. However, it is first important in a book which looks at the various forms of accountability, to explore further the nature of legal accountability and, specifically, to try and distinguish the nurse's legal accountability from other types of accountability.

THE VARIOUS FORMS OF ACCOUNTABILITY

There is no universally agreed definition of the term accountability or a classification of types (Tingle 1990b). Some definitions have been attempted; Tschudin (1992) stated:

'Accountability means not only having to answer for an action when something goes wrong, but it is a continuous process of monitoring how a nurse performs professionally. The responsibility differs in different situations, but there is a need to be aware that one is constantly responsible, and therefore constantly accountable. A distinction needs to be made between legal and moral accountability.'

Lewis and Batey (1982a,b) stated:

'We define accountability...as the fulfilment of a formal obligation to disclose to referent others the purposes, principles, procedures, relationships, results, income, and expenditures for which one has authority...'

These definitions are useful starting points or templates from which to conduct an analysis of the concept of accountability. Defining accountability does seem to be an almost tautological exercise – the concept is a broad one which is, arguably, indefinable. Nevertheless, the exercise of trying is valuable. Thinking at an abstract level does seem to lead to more reflective professional practice: more thought is given to how a job is performed and the personal accountability attached to that job.

An understanding of the concept of accountability can arguably be obtained from an individual's common experiences and general perceptions. All nurses should be able to offer a meaningful 'gut reaction' definition of the concept, and of many others such as responsibility, autonomy, justice, fairness and quality of life. The essential flavour would seem to be that of answerability, i.e. giving a reasoned account for one's own actions or omissions.

Accountable to whom?

Having discussed definitions of accountability it is necessary to deal with the issue of the direction of accountability: to whom are nurses accountable?

Accountability is a multilayered concept. Arguably, a nurse could be accountable to:

- the profession;
- colleagues;
- the patient;
- the employer;
- society;
- a professional regulatory body;
- the law;
- her immediate family;
- herself.

These levels of accountability are not all of equal importance: some are more important than others and conflict between them is certainly possible. A nurse may be asked to work on a ward which is chronically understaffed, but does not say anything about the poor working conditions. As a result of the workload, and doing her best to cope, the nurse injures a patient in the course of administering an intravenous infusion, which a busy doctor had requested and which she was not qualified to do. The nurse knew that she lacked the competence to carry out the procedure but wanted to appear helpful and, being too busy, there was no time to discuss the matter. All the forms of accountability can apply here:

- Patient accountability: The UKCC (1989) would say that the nurse was primarily accountable to the patient.
- Employee accountability: The nurse's employer would say that the nurse is accountable to them as an employee, by virtue of her contract of employment.
- UKCC accountability: The UKCC could view her conduct as being professional misconduct, and disciplinary proceedings could result.

- Society accountability: Society has an interest in the situation, as safe hospitals are clearly in the public interest and furthermore public money from taxes funds the NHS.
- Legal accountability: The nurse owes a personal legal duty of care to the injured patient. The patient could take legal action for compensation for breach of this legal duty. A judge would hear the evidence and the nurse would have to account for both actions and omissions.
- Self-accountability: The negligent nurse also has to live with the decision taken. She has to answer to herself and, if possible, justify the misconduct.
- Professional accountability: Other nurses would seek explanations of this nurse's conduct and, further, they have a duty not to bring the profession into disrepute.
- Colleague accountability: Colleagues would also require an explanation.
- Immediate family accountability: The nurse's immediate family would also be concerned if she was distressed, and would naturally require an explanation. Also, as members of the public, taxpayers and users of the NHS, the immediate family of the patient have a legitimate right to ask questions.

ACCOUNTABILITY AND SANCTIONS

In order to fully understand the different forms of accountability it is necessary to determine the relative weight of each one. Which form of accountability can impose the harshest sanction on the nurse for transgression? What is harsh will necessarily be a value judgement, on which there will be differences of opinion. Logically, harshness can be looked at in terms of the financial and emotional hardship imposed by the accountability body:

- The UKCC can remove the nurse from the register.
- Society, colleagues and family can admonish the nurse.
- The employer can dismiss her.
- She can hate herself.
- The law can punish her by imprisonment or fine, and can award compensation and the costs of the action.

Imprisonment would be the harshest of the sanctions discussed in terms of the emotional and financial hardship imposed. The law is therefore the accountability mechanism that could impose the harshest sanction, and is therefore the one that would have the most direct effect on the nurse.

The nature and application of law and accountability to nursing has been discussed above. In order to further illustrate the nature of legal accountability in a wider health-care context, the issue of the allocation of scarce resources will be discussed. The discussion begins with an analysis of the nurse's role in resource allocation and the conflicts of accountability that can occur.

THE ALLOCATION OF HEALTH-CARE RESOURCES

The nurse's role

The NHS has limited resources to meet a seemingly infinite demand for its services. It is, therefore, an inevitable fact of professional life that decisions have to be made on how best to use these resources (Klein and Redmayne 1992).

Resourcing decisions are made at various levels in nursing, from the charge nurse and their ward budget at one extreme to the Director of Nursing Services at the other. The decisions made will affect everyone concerned with the organization, from staff and patients to suppliers of equipment and services. The reality of budget decision making affects all industries, professions and commercial organizations, as resources are rarely unlimited.

In the context of the NHS, resource issues do generate a lot of publicity and emotive debate. This is understandable, as the issues at stake are health and, sometimes, life (see 'Sick boy seeks court ruling on closure' in *The Times* of 9 June 1993, and 'Kidney patients die as costly dialysis machines lie idle' in *The Times* of 26 July 1993 and Regina v. Cambridge District Health Authority (1995)).

A conflict of accountability

Nurses can experience a conflict of accountability in this area (see Loe 1995). For example, a hospital manager may feel that the staffing level on one ward is just about safe and, therefore, acceptable. No other staff can be obtained because of budget constraints. The manager would like more staff but cannot obtain the necessary extra funding. The nurses on duty are aware of the budget problems but feel that patient safety is being compromised by the poor staffing levels. They are employees, with legal obligations to their employer, and are therefore accountable to them (Tingle 1993b). They are under a legal duty to cooperate with their employer and to obey all reasonable instructions. Employees must also exercise reasonable care and skill in doing their job. The nurses make their views known to management, but management does nothing about it and tells them to carry on as best as they can. The staffing levels remain the same.

The nurses are also accountable to the UKCC and must ensure that they follow their advice in this situation. *The Code of Professional Conduct* (UKCC 1992a) states (clause 12): 'Report to an appropriate person or authority any circumstances in which safe and appropriate care for patients and clients cannot be provided'.

The notion of advocacy by nurses on behalf of patients is also relevant to any consideration of accountability, particularly where conflicts may arise. The UKCC have made nurses primarily accountable to the patient. Section H, Summary of the principles against which to exercise accountability (UKCC 1989), states:

'1. The interests of the patient or client are paramount.
2. Professional accountability must be exercised in such a manner as to ensure that the primacy of the interests of patients or clients is respected and must not be overridden by those of the profession or their practitioners.
3. The exercise of accountability requires the practitioner to seek to achieve and maintain high standards...'

The notion of patient advocacy has, however, been criticized. Allmark and Klarzynski (1992) have argued that the role of nurse is incompatible with that of patient advocate because of the non-mandated nature of the nurse advocate – patients have no choice in who nurses them, and may not wish to be advocated on behalf of – and the fact that the nurse is a member of the health-care team that gives treatment against which the patient may wish to advocate. Furthermore, it has never been clarified what the outcome should be when a nurse takes on the role of patient advocate and thereby comes into conflict with medical staff. Surely both groups would claim to have the best interests of the patient at heart, therefore who is advocating?

THE ROLE OF THE LAW: LEGAL ACCOUNTABILITY

In discussing the problems above there is also the legal accountability of the various parties to consider. The nurses, managers, the employing health authority or NHS Trust all owe the patient a legal duty of care, and all the other mechanisms of accountability discussed earlier will apply. If a patient on the ward suffers an injury which could easily have been avoided had there been adequate staffing levels, then there may be a real possibility of a legal action and legal accountability will have the most direct effect on the parties involved in the case.

It will be recalled that this legal duty is a duty not to expose the patient to unreasonable risks. It requires people to behave reasonably towards their neighbours. A fundamental question will be the extent to which they all did behave reasonably in the circumstances of the case in question.

The nurses, manager and employer could all find themselves in court having to explain themselves. The nurses could even be sued directly by the patient, although it is more likely that their employers would be named in the writ under the principle of vicarious liability discussed earlier. In some circumstances, however, employers could be directly and not vicariously liable to the injured plaintiff (Jones 1991; Old 1993).

A number of court cases (Newdick 1993; Tingle 1992b) have gone to court on the issue of health-care resources and organization, and negligence. A major case is Bull v. Devon Area Health Authority in 1989, reported in the 1993 *Medical Law Report*, **4** p.117. This is a case that has important implications for all health-care professionals.

Organization of services

In the case of the Negligent Organization of Maternity Services: Bull v. Devon Area Health Authority, Mrs Bull went into hospital in premature labour, carrying uniovular twins sharing the same placenta. At 7.27 p.m. the first twin, later named Darryl, was spontaneously delivered and was a male, class A. The second twin, later named Stuart, was delivered 68 minutes later but was subsequently found to have been born with severe brain damage. Stuart should have been delivered as soon as practicable after the first twin and, in any event, within 20 minutes. Specialist medical staff should have attended Mrs Bull in sufficient time to deal with the sort of emergency that arose in the case. Proper assistance was not readily available and the maternity service was found to be negligently organized. Lord Justice Slade stated:

> 'In cases where multiple births were involved, the system in operation at the hospital...was obviously operating on a knife edge. It had to be operated with maximum efficiency.'

This judge was prepared to presume negligence from the facts of the case under a legal principle known as *res ipsa loquitur*. The defendants could not satisfactorily explain the delay in securing specialist medical staff.

Another senior judge, Lord Justice Dillon, stated:

> 'The Exeter City Hospital provides a maternity service for expectant mothers, and any hospital which provides such a service ought to be able to cope with the not particularly out of the way case of a healthy young mother in somewhat premature labour with twins.'

He went on to say that there should have been 'a staff **reasonably sufficient for the foreseeable requirements of the patient'**.

Lord Justice Mustill addressed the hypothetical argument that the hospital providing a public service had done the best it could with the limited resources it had at its disposal:

> 'Again, I have some reservations about this contention, which are not allayed by the submission that hospital medicine is a public service. So it is, but there are other public services in respect of which it is not necessarily an answer to allegations of unsafety that there were insufficient resources to enable the administrators to do everything which they would like to do.'

Damages of £750,000 were later awarded (Miles 1990).

The Bull case shows that the courts are not afraid to grapple with the issue of health-care resources where failure to organize them properly results in negligence. In this case Lord Justice Mustill was not prepared to give the health authority a discount in safety standards because a publicly funded NHS hospital was involved.

Standards of care

Another case which also looks at allegations of negligence and health-care resources and organization is in the context of standards of care for the mentally ill in hospital. Knight and Others v. Home Office and Another, in the 1990 *All England Law Reports* 3 p.237.

Paul Barrington Worrell, aged 21 years, committed suicide by hanging at Brixton prison. He was mentally ill, with known suicidal tendencies, and his personal representatives sued for negligence. A number of allegations were made which included the defendants' failure to provide a proper system, proper staff and facilities for the care of the deceased, and failing to take proper care of his safety. The main thrust of the plaintiffs' case was that the defendants were negligent because the general standard of care provided in the prison was inadequate. The standard of care in the prison hospital should have been the same as that in a psychiatric hospital outside prison, and it fell below that standard. This argument was rejected by the judge and no negligence was found in this case.

Mr Justice Pill stated:

'In making the decision as to the standard to be demanded the court must, however, bear in mind as one factor that resources available for the public service are limited and that the allocation of resources is a matter for parliament...Even in a medical situation outside prison, the standard of care required will vary with the context. The facilities available to deal with an emergency in a general practitioner's surgery cannot be expected to be as ample as those available in the casualty department of a general hospital, for example...The duty is tailored to the act and function to be performed.'

It is possible to agree with Mr Justice Pill's approximation of the standard of care in the case. Prison hospitals and specialist psychiatric hospitals perform different functions with different facilities and missions. However, the judge's reference to public services and parliament's function does cause some concern. The judge did appear to be quite influenced by these factors. His comments are in marked contrast to the sentiments expressed by Lord Justice Mustill in the Bull case and in another case, Wilsher v. Essex Area Health Authority, in the 1986 *All England Law Reports* 3 p.801.

The slippery slope for judges to avoid is that of sanctioning reductions in standards of care in public sector hospitals because parliament controls their resources and these are limited. All hospitals open for public service should provide, in Lord Justice Dillon's words from the Bull case, '**a staff reasonably sufficient for the foreseeable requirements of the patient**'. Lack of resources should not prevent the reasonable and safe provision of treatment. A hospital unit or ward which cannot provide 'a staff reasonably sufficient for the foreseeable requirements of the patient' should, arguably, close until it is able to do so, otherwise a potentially negligent health-care system is *prima facie* in operation.

The managers and staff are between a rock and a hard place in this situation. There are no easy answers to the problem.

This discussion has focused on the area where it has been alleged that there was negligence in resource organization and allocation which resulted in patient injury (Jones 1991). The term 'health-care resource' has a wide meaning and includes medical and nursing staff as well as plant and equipment.

There are other cases that have been brought by patients who have had to wait a long time for urgent treatment because a hospital could not help them due to limited resources. The courts have displayed a cautious attitude in these cases.

Obligation to treat

The courts will not review or challenge a health authority's or even a doctor's decision not to treat unless the decision was so unreasonable that no reasonable health authority or doctor would have made such a decision in the circumstances of the case, or where there was a breach of public law duties. The courts do not want to be used to organize hospital waiting lists and to set new hospital spending priorities. Quite understandably, they do not want to take upon themselves the role of arbiters of social policy. Some of these cases will now be discussed.

Hole in the heart baby requires operation: re Walker's application, in *The Times Law Report* (26 November 1987), describes how necessary heart surgery was postponed on five occasions because of a lack of specially trained nurses and accompanying facilities which did not allow the expansion of the intensive care unit. The baby was under no immediate risk but the mother sought to challenge in court the health authority's decision to postpone the operation, through a legal process known as judicial review. She failed in her action. The senior appeal court judge, Sir John Donaldson, as he then was, stated:

> '...that it was not for the court to interfere and substitute its own judgement for that of those responsible for the allocation of resources. It would only interfere if there had been a failure to allocate funds in a way which was 'unreasonable'...or where there were breaches of public-law duties.'

On similar facts the Court of Appeal in R. v. Central Birmingham Health Authority *ex parte* Collier 1988, Unreported, in Lexis Transcript (1988, Butterworths Telepublishing, London) dismissed a similar application and the principles in the earlier Walker case were said to apply even where there was an immediate danger to health.

Another perspective to the resource allocation issue can be seen in the case of Re J. (1992). J. was 16 months old and was severely mentally and physically handicapped. He sustained his injuries as a result of hitting his head in an accidental fall when he was 4 weeks old. He suffered from severe cerebral palsy, epilepsy and cortical blindness. He had to be fed via a nasogastric tube. Parental responsibility for him was shared between his parents and the local authority. He was placed with foster parents. There was unanimous medical opinion that he was unlikely to develop beyond his present level of functioning and that that level might deteriorate. He would have a short life. Twenty-four-hour attention and regular medication was required. The consultant paediatrician in charge of his case made two reports, which included a statement that it would not be medically appropriate to intervene with intensive therapeutic measures such as artificial ventilation if the child were to suffer a life-threatening event.

The child's mother and the local authority sought a court order that the health authority continue to provide all available treatment to J., including 'intensive resuscitation'. Their application did not succeed. The court would not require a doctor to follow a particular course of treatment against their best professional judgement.

Lord Donaldson, the senior appeal court judge, did comment on the issue of health-care resources when he was considering the errors of the judge who first tried the case in the lower court, and who had made an interim injunctive order which the Court of Appeal set aside.

In discussing the judge's order he stated:

> '...it does not adequately take account of the sad fact of life that health authorities may on occasion find that they have too few resources, either human or material or both, to treat all the patients whom they would like to treat in the way which they would like to treat them. It is then their duty to make choices. The court, when considering what course to adopt in relation to a particular child, has no knowledge of competing claims to a health authority's resources and is in no position to express any view as to how it should elect to deploy them.'

The judges in this case were faced with competing interests and they made choices which they justified. They played a very important role in health-care resource decision making by resolving the dispute, and set out legal principles which will apply in these types of case in the future. A key legal principle in Re J. was that the professional judgement of the medical practitioner was to be respected; a point also reinforced in Regina v. Cambridge Health Authority, *ex parte* B (1995) [discussed in *Health Care Risk Reports*, **1**: 5 (1995) 3].

CONCLUSION

It is possible to see some mixed messages coming from the courts when all the health-care resource allocation cases are considered together. The courts appear to be treading very carefully, but will not be afraid to challenge a decision in appropriate circumstances.

Health-care resource allocators must act reasonably to be within the law. The concept of reasonableness does, however, allow them a fair degree of latitude in their decision making. It would be difficult, although not impossible, to imagine a health authority making a health-care resource allocation decision that was so unreasonable that no reasonable health authority would have made it.

The courts do maintain an important potential to safeguard patient's rights and interests in the NHS. They resolve disputes when called upon to do so, and through that process set legal principles which provide a broad framework for health-care resource allocation. Health-care resource allocators are legally accountable for their decision making.

Accountability – the ethical dimension

11

Kath Melia

INTRODUCTION

Accountability is an important concept in a health-care system which sets great store by efficiency, quality and audit. As in other areas of public service, accountability has become a commonplace in any discussion about professional activity. The reasons for this go beyond the relatively simple notion of accountability as in lines of accountability and management structures. Professions have been accorded a position of trust in society, and are therefore obliged to account for themselves and to demonstrate that they do not, and will not, abuse that public trust. Any group which provides a complex service for society does so through a bureaucratic organizational structure in which roles and lines of accountability are clearly defined. Nurses as a professional group present perhaps one of the most complex organizational challenges for the new-style management-oriented health service because nursing has a strong line management culture yet has to find a means of functioning in the world of directorates. The managerial approach to the organization of health care is a pragmatic one, necessitated by the fact that it involves large numbers of strangers providing a comprehensive and integrated service for even larger numbers of strangers.

ORGANIZATION OF NURSING

Health-care professionals organize themselves along bureaucratic lines, and nursing in particular has long had a system of line management following on from its history of authority in religious and military communities. It seems, then, natural enough to want to discuss accountability in the context of nursing because line management works precisely through lines of accountability. The question we have to ask is, why is it of any interest in a moral sense? In the bureaucratic organizational chart that shows us who is accountable to whom for what, is there anything that might give rise to ethical questions? Before asserting that there are ethical issues to be considered when we think about accountability, we need to stop and think what these might be.

If accountability means liable to account, to give a reason or explanation, or to answer as one responsible, then there seems to be nothing ethically problematic about it. These are organizational rather than ethical issues. Why, therefore, did it seem so obvious from the outset and why, indeed, did it seem to the editor of this volume that ethics has a place here? If accountability has to do with flowcharts and the question of who reports to whom, then there may be problems, but they are likely to be organizational ones or issues of power, not ethics.

If, however, we think about the individual who is accountable to X for something or other, what that individual has is responsibility for that for which they are accountable. In the area of responsibility there are indeed ethical issues, nay minefields. Responsibility is about being called to account, being responsible, being accountable for one's actions and being a free moral agent. It is this freedom of moral agency during the space of time when an individual is carrying out the activities for which he or she is accountable that is of real interest in terms of an ethical debate. The notion of accountability provides the form, the bureaucratic wiring diagram for the delivery of the service. The content or the quality of the activities that are carried out as part of the service depend upon the responsibility that the individual takes for the action.

RESPECT FOR PERSONS

In the exercise of responsibility in the context of nursing it seems clear that two of the basic underlying principles are those of respect for persons and beneficence. The individual nurse, and sometimes the patient involved, will often be the only people with a clear idea of the nature of much of the care given. In terms of accountability it can be said that so many patients have been bathed, fed, given medication or whatever, but little more can be known about the nature of the activity. If we become interested in the notion of responsibility, it does not necessarily make the care any more publicly known, but it does open up a different agenda. To talk about being responsible for a patient does, I would argue, bring into sharper focus the moral agenda and leads us to consider the issues involved. I would not seek to push the distinction between accountability and responsibility much further, as it then becomes no more than a question of semantics. It is, however, interesting to note that in some languages, for instance Spanish, there is no separate word for accountability: it is all 'responsibility'. In English there may be two words and endless fine details in the definition, but the argument and the difficulty, I would suggest, come with responsibility.

The degree of responsibility that individual nurses carry will vary with seniority, experience and organizational factors. It is, nevertheless, possible to consider responsibility in broad terms which could be said to be universally applicable. If we take the basic principles mentioned above, respect for persons and beneficence, we can start from the premise that nurses, in exercising their responsibility for patient care, will be concerned to do good and prevent harm and to respect the autonomy of the individual patient. Fine words, and little to object to, but when we consider the social context in which nursing care is delivered we have to consider the complexities of the situation. How do we know what patients want? How do nurses carry their responsibility to act according to the principle of beneficence when a patient's own wishes might run counter to their interests? What exactly does responsibility mean?

REALMS OF RESPONSIBILITY

It is perhaps helpful to think of responsibility in terms of different levels or realms of responsibility (Thompson *et al.* 1994). Nurses are responsible for their own actions, both morally and legally. Responsibility, in moral terms, is a burden that comes with taking up nursing as an occupation. Decisions that we make about how we care for patients, how much of our time and selves we put into the work, and what quality of care we offer are rather individualistic and in many ways known only to the individual nurse and patients concerned. If nurses are to be responsible for the care they give, they have to keep themselves informed of advances in practice. It is also the case that individual nurses have a responsibility to play their part in the advancement of nursing knowledge. Not every nurse will be engaged in research, but precise and accurate record keeping will assist in the evaluation of practice and form part of the wider enterprise of nursing research. In order to practise nursing in a morally acceptable way nurses must be satisfied that they are working according to the latest available knowledge and playing their part in input to the development of that knowledge. Nurses have a personal responsibility to keep themselves updated in this way.

At another level there is what is known as fiduciary responsibility, that is, when someone is entrusted to the care of another. This is common in nursing, when patients cannot be said to be in control of their lives, for instance children, the mentally ill or incompetent and, of course, the unconscious. The fiduciary responsibility that the nurse takes on in these situations is based on the moral authority that comes from the trust society or the individual patient has placed in the nursing profession. This brings us to a third type of responsibility, that is, responsibility for one's practice as a member of the nursing profession. Professional groups have a degree of control over their work and to some extent determine what will be its nature. As members of a publicly recognized and trusted professional group, individual nurses have a responsibility to their profession. The profession's code of ethics, in this case the *Code of Professional Conduct* (UKCC 1992a), is the means by which the profession publicly proclaims its trustworthiness. In other words, the professional code serves as a guide to practice which is accepted by the profession as a whole, rather than leaving members to follow their own moral codes. It also provides a means of indicating to the society served by the profession that these are the principles according to which nurses practice.

Being responsible to a profession, and practising according to an agreed professional morality rather than following individual moral codes, has its attractions but also gives rise to difficulties when individual nurses find that their personal morality is at odds with the professional code. Responsibility in its widest sense is the responsibility that nurses have to the society in which they practise. As Thompson points out:

'As a professional member of the NHS staff, the nurse has responsibility for maintaining the general standards of nursing care. As members of a profession committed to the care of patients, nurses have responsibilities to influence health policy and the allocation of resources. Nurses are public officers, even public servants, with both civic and political duties. They have individual civic responsibility to society to draw attention to specific examples of incompetence, or negligence or where standards of care have become unacceptable' (Thompson *et al.* 1994).

CONCLUSION

This responsibility to the public is perhaps the most difficult to adopt. Although it does not necessarily arise as an everyday issue, it may well be difficult for nurses to act in accordance with it if they have to consider their responsibility for the interests of individual patients against their responsibility for groups of patients. The inclination of individual nurses to act in a particular way has to be weighed in the light of the demands made upon them by the Trust or the union, or indeed the health-care team within which they are working. Having a responsibility to society while caring for particular individuals has its challenges. As budgets are devolved to units the balance that has to be found between the best for an individual and the best for the patient/client group as a whole comes ever closer to the 'careplace', as it were. This brings into clear view the long-standing moral dilemma which the utilitarians attempt to solve by the 'greatest good for the greatest number' approach. Utilitarianism notoriously leaves the individual in the background, and it is only when we think in terms of respect for persons that the individual comes to the fore. Then the long-standing ethical debate about the rights of the individual versus the rights of the group, or indeed society, takes on real meaning.

Accountability in life and death decisions

12

Hazel McHaffie

INTRODUCTION

'Any man's death diminishes me because I am involved in Mankind.'

John Donne's immortal words capture the essential pain of death: it is something which affects us all profoundly. It is natural to try to avoid addressing the issues associated with mortality and loss. Society itself has thrown a circle of taboos around the subject.

Nurses, of course, confront dying in a way that the general public do not: it is part of their professional lives. Even so, there is a real sense in which nurses do make determined and frequent attempts to resist its impact. Some choose specialties where patients seldom die; others spend their working hours fighting to extend the lives of the terminally ill; almost all, when faced with a sudden collapse, will seek fiercely to prevent the patient from dying. Losing the battle is undoubtedly a painful and emotional experience, particularly where the life has been short and the death is perceived as tragic. I have personally heard and felt this pain acutely in the areas of neonatal intensive care and HIV/AIDS, where babies and young people die fairly frequently. Simply being caught up in the powerful feelings associated with such losses can obscure clear thinking. Nurses are not, and nor should they be, automata.

Not only are efforts made to avoid the emotional impact in clinical practice, but nurses have traditionally taken a back seat when it comes to decision-making in relation to prolonging life and assisting death. These matters have been perceived as lying almost exclusively in the doctors' domain. Given the vital role of nurses in the care of patients, however, it is entirely inappropriate for them to abdicate responsibility in this way. Such weighty decisions are not the proper burden of a single individual. There needs to be a combination of many perspectives. The different disciplines are closely interwoven and their roles and responsibilities overlap. Nurses, then, must think through the issues carefully and calmly.

To be truly accountable is to be able to defend one's actions. Clearly, the same fundamental issues which are enshrined in codes of conduct apply in the care of patients and relatives in this as in every other area of practice. Rather than reiterating the minutiae of accountability in a practical sense, this discussion will concentrate on the arguments which underpin any decision to prolong a life or assist a death. It is in fully thinking through the meaning, implications and consequences of these arguments that nurses will be able to defend the course of action taken and be properly accountable for their practice. These are not academic points: they affect real people. They have direct and sobering effects on the patient, the relatives, and also the carers. All too often the case is presented for one side or another with almost no reference to alternative perspectives or pragmatic considerations. Nurses must challenge received wisdom when it comes to matters of life or death, taking full account not only of basic ethical principles but also of duties and responsibilities, of the long-term as well as the short-term consequences of these awesome decisions.

THE PRESENT POSITION

In the past, fear of retribution and a sense that decisions relating to prolonging life are private, have forced doctors into covert practices without the benefit of support from, or discussion with, colleagues. It is known nowadays that there is widespread agreement among doctors with the idea of helping to end suffering. Indeed, Dr Richard Smith, editor of the *British Medical Journal*, has gone so far as to say that most doctors have hastened the deaths of some of their patients (Smith 1993). Where individuals have been brave enough to declare their hand, however, there has been a price to pay and a few have faced prosecution on criminal charges. Small wonder, then, that most keep quiet about what they do. Even today, in The Netherlands, where the practice of euthanasia is not punishable provided certain clear guidelines are followed, there is widespread under-reporting of medical involvement (Borst-Eilers 1993). Fear of the law, however, does not constitute an ethical reason to treat or not to treat, even though it may well be a motivating factor. It is imperative that these issues are dealt with openly and honestly.

Traditionally, doctors have been largely left to practise as they saw fit, but their paternalistic traditions have been seriously challenged in recent years:

'Philosophers have moved into medicine in force in the past 10 years, making doctors think much more clearly about how they take ethical decisions. The paternalist tradition that doctors know best has begun to crumble under this onslaught: there have to be very cogent reasons for overriding patient autonomy. This ethical analysis has come at the same time as a consumer tide which insists that the patient rather than the professional be in charge' (Smith 1993).

If Shaw's dictum that all professions are conspiracies against the laity is to be taken seriously, then this scrutiny of medical and nursing practice must, in the end, be strengthening for health-care professionals, even though at the time it might feel very uncomfortable. Examination and questioning by those who have never been clinically involved in these agonizing decisions may be viewed with some dismay: how can they understand the skilled judgements and fine nuances? But some can comprehend the legal niceties, the philosophical distinctions and the family implications far better than the doctors and nurses. Combined thinking from different perspectives has the potential to improve rather than undermine professional decision-making. Such open debate would have been almost unthinkable even 30 years ago; today it has become a necessity.

Recent cases have hit the headlines and taken these matters out of the professional closet. They are seen as real issues and part of the working lives of practising doctors and nurses. Public scrutiny, on the one hand, has led to a greater imperative to tell the truth. On the other hand, it has also underlined the tension between private troubles and public issues. Some individuals have paid a high price for these decisions to move into a wider arena and be openly debated. An examination of two of them will help to underline the relevance of a discussion of these issues.

Dr Nigel Cox

Dr Nigel Cox is a consultant rheumatologist in Winchester. For 13 years he had cared for a patient, Mrs Lillian Boyes, who suffered from acute rheumatoid arthritis. In 1992 she was 70 years of age and in excruciating pain, with ulcers and abscesses on her legs and arms, a rectal sore which penetrated to the bone, fractured vertebrae and gangrene from her treatment with steroids. She would scream in agony if touched and morphine in increasing doses gave her no relief. Both she and her sons appealed for her to be helped to die. Initially her request was refused, but eventually Dr Cox administered a lethal injection of potassium chloride. It was a few days later that a nurse, Sister Roisin Hart, discovered his action recorded in Mrs Boyes' notes, and felt she had no alternative but to report him.

Questions were inevitably raised about the judgement of one doctor. A specific criticism levelled at Dr Cox was his failure to apply to other experts in the field of palliative care (St John-Smith and Edwards 1992). Following the General Medical Council's professional conduct committee's decision not to impose disciplinary sanctions on him, his employing authority agreed to his return to work on certain conditions. He was to take part in meetings arranged by managers 'to explore problems and build relationships'; to have a senior consultant as his mentor; and be attached to a palliative unit in order 'to become familiar with the full range of techniques' (Dyer 1992). The health authority recognized the potential difficulties for Dr Cox and his colleagues in his return to work following the court case and disciplinary hearing.

Whereas Dr Cox was convicted and his judgement questioned, the action of Sister Hart was commended. She had 'courageously followed' her professional code of practice 'with absolute integrity' (Dyer 1992). At the very least, this case has revealed a failure of communication. That it became necessary for one professional to report another in this serious way exposes the weaknesses in a system which has not taken account of the different opinions and beliefs of the various individuals most closely involved. We shall return to the issues this case highlights: the contribution of the law, the adequacy of professional codes, the euthanasia debate, underlying ethical issues and conflicts between professionals.

Tony Bland

Tony Bland was a 17-year-old football fan crushed during the Hillsborough disaster at the FA Cup semifinal in April 1989, at which 95 other people died. Tony did not die at the time but his injuries were so severe that he never regained consciousness, and a persistent vegetative state was eventually diagnosed. In time, Tony's parents and medical attendants came to believe that there was no merit in continuing to prolong his life, since the overwhelming medical evidence was that he would never recover or improve. A prolonged legal battle ensued as appeals were made to the High Court and the House of Lords. It took 3 years, fierce public debate and much agonizing on everyone's part in order to arrive at a decision that his feeding tube could be removed and he could be allowed to die. This was not a matter of switching off a ventilator or withdrawing other extraordinary life-saving measures, it was a matter of simply not feeding him.

As well as raising sensitive issues relating to matters of treatment, personhood and sentience, this case brought to the fore the debate about responsibility. Part of the unease arose from the feeling that the law was deciding what doctors could or could not do. It emerged during this appeal that a number of patients in a persistent vegetative state had died without appeal or fuss in Scotland, and that the variations in the law were confounding. The Law Lords accepted that the Tony Bland case challenged ideas of the sanctity of life; a duty to care on the part of doctors; the best interest of the patient; and the ethical difference between withdrawing treatment and active euthanasia. They concluded that their decision was for this case alone and that it would probably 'emphasize the distortions of a legal structure which is already both morally and intellectually misshapen' (House of Lords 1993).

This case, like the Cox one, exposed the tension between public interest and private grief. Doctor James Howe, who was the consultant in charge of Tony Bland, was forced into the public eye. His appeal requesting the courts to decide followed a statement by the local coroner that withdrawing treatment would result in prosecution. It is not surprising that he had no appetite for making the decision sensitively, quietly and autonomously. To do so could have protected both himself and the parents from public scrutiny and vilification, but laid him open to a charge of murder. He was caught on a knife-edge between the personal distress of all concerned with this patient's plight and possible criminal charges. But in this case there was no whistle blowing – he himself brought the case to the courts. Indeed, he repeatedly paid tribute to the nurses caring for Tony, and the devotion of the young man's parents. Fundamental issues were exposed for scrutiny by this case. Modern technology and medical advances have now blurred the edges which distinguish life from death (Lamb 1985).

'Death has become a great uncertainty for us, at both the conceptual and public policy levels. Some uncertainties are tolerable; others are not. Since dying and death are sources of the deepest, most intractable anguish that humans can suffer, uncertainty here is morally intolerable, for it promises only to compound that anguish, not diminish it' (Gervais 1986).

With the Tony Bland case the demarcations were further questioned, the debates about euthanasia and withdrawal of treatment were revisited, quality of life issues re-emerged and principles of distributive justice took on poignant significance. We shall return to these issues later. One thing that these two cases has demonstrated is that decisions may depend more on the physician's own values and willingness to take risks than on the exact nature of the patient's or relatives' request. Due to the fact that other choices regarding treatment or no treatment are less conspicuous than those directly addressing the hastening of death, they are less subject to control and review. This means that they are more open to abuse and idiosyncratic decision-making. It can, unfortunately, also mean that in some cases patients are forced to die alone, or relatives and friends are left to shoulder an immense personal burden, to protect others from legal peril. There is no easy answer: the essential debate must be firmly rooted in the realities of actual day-to-day practice in medicine and nursing:

'We cannot resolve these moral tensions by making one side of the tension disappear. Instead, we must learn to live with these tensions within a pluralistic society. This requires more reliance on negotiation, compromise, and practical reasoning, and less on abstract ethical theory' (Brody 1992).

Not all cases are extreme or bizarre. There are far fewer cases of fetuses being kept alive in brain-dead mothers (as reported in *Der Spiegel* during 1992) than there are severely impaired infants being born. Persistent vegetative state affects many fewer people than dementia, but the decisions relating to life and death are painful and complex in most of these situations. What is the nurse's responsibility in all of this? They are, after all, accountable in law to their profession, to their patients and relatives, and to themselves. If they hold a religious belief, they also feel accountable to a higher authority.

THE LEGAL BOUNDARIES

The law, as it stands, is unequivocal: to kill a living person deliberately is murder. This prohibition is based on the fundamental belief that human life is sacred. Recognized exceptions spring instantly to mind which cast doubt on whether the sanctity of life is in reality treated as a moral absolute – self-defence, so-called just wars and capital punishment, to name the most obvious. The judgements in cases where lay people have assisted suicide or performed euthanasia in cases of intractable pain, or where doctors have withheld treatment or hastened death in some way bear testament to the unease which society feels about the grey area between deliberate killing and the merciful easing of suffering.

Up until 1961 suicide was illegal in the UK, and it is still illegal to assist suicide or to commit euthanasia. But modern technology and scientific advances sometimes produce dilemmas and force relatives and friends into intolerable corners. Do the professionals who control these things not have a concomitant responsibility to provide a way out when medicine can do no more to help a person live well? Some bolder individuals have felt strongly enough about the subject to go public over their own role in assisting death (for example Duff and Campbell 1973; Humphries 1978; and a current (1995) case of a Dutch paediatrician whose actions are making legal history because he officially recorded his active role in the death of a baby).

It is important to emphasize that, just because something is illegal, it is not necessarily morally wrong. Conversely, because something is legal it does not mean that it is necessarily morally right. Thus, many would argue that though abortion is legal it is in the majority of cases morally indefensible: a law can be introduced because it offers the better of two undesirable alternatives. The British system of justice is such that we like to have our laws and our moral standards as nearly equivalent as possible. But sometimes there are compromises: for example, we permit legalized abortion, which most would agree is essentially an undesirable practice, in order to reduce subsequent death and morbidity.

Periodically, anomalies in the law challenge the status quo and force people to look again at whether the law coincides with today's thinking. The Cox and Bland cases challenged thinking about the prolongation of life. Even so, the conclusion of the Law Commission was that:

'...a doctor, however well intentioned, who does a positive act intended to end the life of a patient commits a serious criminal offence, even if the patient requests such steps. However, capable patients are entitled to refuse any treatment, and doctors may withhold or withdraw treatment which is not in the best interests of their patient without being in breach of duty or in breach of the criminal law. This is so even if death is the inevitable consequence' (Law Commission 1993).

The law, then, is 'the codification of the will of the people' (Smith 1992), and where there is too great a tension between a legal verdict and the thinking of the people the law must be reconsidered.

Anyone who has been involved in caring for patients where these agonizing decisions have had to be made, knows the trauma that accompanies the process. Not only the families, but professionals too, agonize and grieve. The various arguments need to be endlessly rehearsed, intimate issues are exposed to fairly public scrutiny, and the final decision carries a heavy weight of responsibility which is apt to resurrect deep emotions long after the event. Involving the courts in these painful decisions troubles many people. Legislation is simply too blunt an instrument to deal with such delicate matters, which affect each person differently. Moreover, if a health-care system is to function well it is essential that the basic trust between patients, their relatives, and doctors and nurses is not eroded; it is too important and too fragile to be exposed to the strain of public and impersonal exposure. This is not to say that patients and their relatives need to place implicit faith in the professions: a healthy dose of scepticism and inquiry can be good, both empowering lay people and keeping the professionals alert to their responsibilities.

It can therefore be argued that society may healthily challenge but should not, without strong reason, dictate to doctors and nurses. Their expertise and ethical awareness should permit them to make appropriate choices and guide patients and relatives wisely, lawfully and morally. However, this places a grave responsibility on health-care workers. As we have seen, in some instances decisions are at the very least questionable. Who will patrol the corridors to ensure that standards are maintained? Can we be sure that this internal autonomy is not going to lead to an avalanche of idiosyncratic abuse of power? Just how are practitioners accountable to their profession?

PROFESSIONAL ACCOUNTABILITY

Almost inevitably, when the accountability of doctors is considered, their allegiance to the Hippocratic Oath is cited as a failsafe mechanism to guard against illegal or immoral practice. Where they deviate from the accepted path there is a disciplinary procedure dictated by the General Medical Council, with their peers leading an internal enquiry. This has all the advantages of those well versed in the nuances and realities of medical practice considering the issues from an informed and experienced angle. It does, however, raise questions in the public mind about whether the profession closes ranks and whether justice will be done.

Nursing is rather different in its code of practice. Early nursing codes reflected the idea of nursing as being subservient to medicine: 'The nurse is under obligation to carry out the physician's orders intelligently and loyally' (International Council of Nurses 1965). But by the early 1990s this became 'or in a collaborative and cooperative manner with health-care professionals and others involved in providing care, and recognize and respect their particular contributions within the care team' (UKCC 1992a).

Responsibility is placed fairly and squarely with nurses, who are personally accountable for their actions and behaviours. In the exercise of this accountability nurses are instructed to 'act always in such a manner as to promote and safeguard the interests and wellbeing of patients', and to 'ensure that no action or omission', either on their own part or within their sphere of responsibility, 'is detrimental to the interests, condition or safety of patients'. And here we begin to see potential for conflict. For all these sentiments are, it seems, open to either a narrow or a more liberal interpretation.

A direct injunction in the UKCC Code of Conduct to 'report to an appropriate person or authority, having regard to the physical, psychological and social effects on patients and clients, any circumstances in the environment of care which could jeopardize standards of practice' presumably led Sister Roisin Hart to report her colleague, Dr Nigel Cox. She was commended by her health authority for her professional response, and the integrity with which she followed her code of conduct. Presumably there was a failure to 'work in a collaborative and cooperative manner' with colleagues which led to the action in the first place. Little was said publicly of the relationships existing in the team and it would be inappropriate for outsiders to apportion blame. Rather, this case highlights the need for codes and guidelines to be used intelligently and critically. There is a certain sense of 'being covered' and 'immune to prosecution' if one slavishly follows prescribed rules. Each nurse must, rather, look seriously at what the Codes really mean and question their practice honestly and humbly. A further question which has to be asked is, how well do nurses know their codes? In one study in the USA, none of the 27 nurses interviewed knew the content of their professional code (Davis 1991). Their ethical decision-making was based on clinical experience, personal values and beliefs.

The importance the professions as a whole attach to resolving moral conflicts in the matter of life and death decisions is demonstrated by the recent publication of position documents such as *Resuscitation: Right or Wrong? The moral and legal issues faced by health care professionals* (Royal College of Nursing 1992) and *Cardiopulmonary Resuscitation: A statement from the BMA and RCN* (British Medical Association and Royal College of Nursing 1993). These publications recognize the impossibility of giving definitive judgements for specific situations; instead, they give guidelines on the questions to ask, the factors to balance and the moral concerns that must be considered.

Codes of conduct and professional statements only take us so far. Nurses need to be tested in the fire of real-life dilemmas in order to understand the agony of situation-based ethical decision-making. Moreover, ethical problems in nursing do not present themselves in an orderly, systematic fashion allowing the straightforward application of absolute principles and the following of set guidelines. Each of us brings something of our own history, experiences, beliefs and values to any given situation. It is important to stress that:

'Ethical behavior is not the display of one's moral rectitude in times of crisis. It is the day-by-day expression of one's commitment to other persons and the ways in which human beings relate to one another in their daily interactions' (Levine 1990).

Although the frequency with which we each have to address the issues relating to life and death decisions is not great, nevertheless, when these situations do arise the consequences are momentous and far-reaching.

As we have already said, in all of our deliberations about these issues it is essential to keep them firmly rooted in the practical disciplines of medicine and nursing. It is relatively easy to debate the arguments for and against things like infertility treatment, abortion and euthanasia in the abstract. Confronted by a distressed person caught in a complex web of divided loyalties and conflicting circumstances, facing a potentially irreversible decision, the issues are not nearly so straightforward.

We can, of course, to some extent use vicarious experience. Imagining ourselves in the position of Sister Roisin Hart or Mrs Boyes or Dr Nigel Cox can help us to explore our own attitudes and beliefs. Programmes such as the Channel 4 series 'Decisions Decisions', with its accompanying booklet (Kelleher 1993), enable us to see in a variety of real-life situations the struggle to decide, the cost to individuals, the conflicts of obligations and the incompatibility of different important duties.

Moral conflict, as a central aspect of human life, can potentially be experienced in a variety of circumstances all of which would not affect any one individual in real life. The very realness of the experiences of ordinary people facing extraordinary choices underlines the fact that more than one course of action can be morally right in any given situation. If we are honestly appraising these situations and weighing up the potential burdens and benefits attending each of the choices, we come some way towards recognizing the real dilemmas. We hear and feel the compelling arguments on both sides (McHattie 1994).

What, then, are the main issues that impinge on nurses in relation to life and death decisions? In reality, it is often difficult to separate the actual act from the consequences or to be sure on which side of the equation death itself comes. Reared in the tradition that death is the ultimate form of consumer resistance (Illich 1977), nurses can sometimes equate dying with failure. Examples of elderly patients being unceremoniously subjected to all the undignified rigours of enthusiastic resuscitation, vividly portray the profession's commitment to life at almost any cost. In the interests of compassion, it is necessary to recognize that in certain circumstances death will best serve the interests of a patient. Can we accurately determine what these circumstances are?

First we will look at the issues which underpin the debate, the arguments relating to whether or not to treat, and whether or not to help to die both being aspects of the same coin. In different circumstances both withholding treatment and administering accepted medical treatment can hasten death: it does not necessarily require the active administration of a lethal substance to help someone to die.

ARGUMENTS FOR HASTENING DEATH

Rights

Various writers and philosophers have attempted to identify the rights of individuals which need to be considered in any dealings with a patient. Lists include the right to be treated in his or her best interests; to a dignified life; to choose between treatment and non-treatment; to cessation of treatment where the burdens substantially outweigh the benefits; to the relief of pain. Acceding to these might entail variously offering or withholding treatment, or managing the case in such a way that death is hastened. But are these rights inviolable? What of the doctors' and nurses' rights? Do they not have the right to act in accordance with professional standards; to refrain from treating or acting in anything to which they have a conscientious objection? What of the rights of other interested parties to assist in the decisions about the best interest of the relative or friend for whom they care? What of the rights of society to determine how far the interests and competing rights of various kinds of patient can be met? For each of these rights there could be set out a responsibility or a duty, but this side of the equation is far less frequently acknowledged. If a patient has a right to demand an end to his suffering, where does the responsibility lie to carry out the appropriate measures?

An extension of modern medicine

Of course, medicine cannot abdicate responsibility for what it has produced. Not only have scientific advances enabled effective cures to be found for most illnesses, but vigorous applications of science have produced tragic situations where lives are saved at the expense of dignity and quality. It is necessary only to look at cases such as Nancy Cruzan, a victim of a car accident (Angell 1990), and Tony Bland, whose case we have already discussed, both of whom were left in a persistent vegetative state; or at baby Andrew Stinson, who endured months of unproductive therapy in his few short months of life (Stinson and Stinson 1983), to acknowledge the responsibility of technological successes. Indeed, it has been pointed out that a tragic irony of our times is that some people now fear living more than dying because they live in dread of becoming prisoners of technology (Angell 1990).

To an extent, the call for help in dying is a response to modern 'high tech' medicine – the last and most compassionate and fair treatment a doctor can give his suffering patient. In reality, it is probable that only a tiny number of doctors would work actively to end the life of a patient, whereas selective non-treatment and hastening death through the application of compassionate relief of suffering are widely practised. It is generally held that allowing someone to die is morally preferable to actively killing them. There are, however, those who say that any distinction between a commission and an omission to act when both have the same effect is an illusion, since the responsibility and the intention are the same (Kuhse 1984; Gillon 1986). Even though they acknowledge that their reasons for holding this view may be tenuous, some doctors will steadfastly maintain that there is a distinction in practice for them:

'Our gut intuition tells us that there is a difference between active and passive euthanasia and we are not going to be browbeaten into changing our minds by mere logic' (Brewin 1986).

In reality, of course, even this distinction is often blurred. Omissions can be active decisions and, indeed, can involve positive actions. An additional aspect of this argument is that merely being passive and allowing nature to take its course can involve the patient in a slow, painful or undignified death.

Eugenics

It would be wrong to omit the argument of eugenics from a consideration of this topic. Some would contend that society has an obligation to eliminate the physically or mentally unfit. Lest we dismiss this argument too summarily on the grounds that it offends our sensibilities, let us not draw a veil over the countless lives which are sacrificed every year in the form of aborted, malformed fetuses. Is it really any different to consider an unborn child to be unfit to live and to deem a teenager in a persistent vegetative state or an adult irreversibly damaged by a cerebrovascular accident to be equally better dead?

Resources

It is a harsh reality that, as society is currently organized, resources are finite. Many of us feel profoundly uneasy when arguments to do with economics enter into those related to the treatment of human beings. However, the principle of distributive justice cannot be ignored. The concept involves examining those factors which will constitute the common good alongside considerations about the specific welfare of one individual or group. All too often, the allocation of resources to one deprives another.

Chancing all on a slim possibility of success may be exciting; the thrill of new developments, of pitting one's wits against the greatest enemy cannot be denied. And after all, heart/lung transplants make the headlines; hernia repairs do not. When we consider the definite good those same resources would produce if used in less heroic procedures, we have to stop and consider. The money spent to send one small girl to America for a rare multiple-organ transplant which might save her life, could buy many hip replacements and certainly give a good quality of life to many suffering adults. For the parents of that little girl, however, her life is precious beyond all other considerations. The doctor or nurse relating to that parent and seeing the private and personal anguish is caught up in the dilemma. It is no longer an academic point. In addition, funds available for one purpose are not necessarily transferrable to another.

Maintaining patients who are in a persistent vegetative state is immensely costly. Can such a cost be justified? To take an extreme case, the longest-known survivor in such a state was a 1-year-old girl who survived an anaesthetic accident and existed for a further 37 years, unknowing and unfeeling (McWhirter 1981). Viewed in the cold light of a retrospective day, such a decision has to be questionable.

ARGUMENTS AGAINST HASTENING DEATH

Sanctity of life

Probably the most powerful argument rehearsed against ending a life is that of the sanctity of life. Those with a religious belief propound the idea that life itself is given by God, and man may not either take it away from another nor hand his own life back when he has had enough of living. It is also an argument used by those who do not hold any belief in a divine creator. A utilitarian argument can be founded on the thesis that if life may be taken, the good of society will be threatened and possibly destroyed. As we have already discussed, there are recognized cases in which lives are taken with the sanction of society and the law. It seems dubious reasoning to defend the execution of a convicted criminal or the slaughter of many innocent civilians in the course of a so-called 'just' war, but to deplore the ending of a life of pain and distress for a person who wishes it, simply on the basis that life is sacred, when in the first case the criminal and the war victims want to live and in the second case the patient wants to die. No-one gets what they want!

If we pursue the argument that life is given by God, we can soon perceive another weakness in the logic. Simply treating patients to prolong their life by any medical intervention, no matter how small, could be seen as 'playing God'. Taking the argument to its logical extreme, if God intended humans to die early of ruptured appendices and pneumonia we should not use our modern skills to restore them to perfect health. These instances of intervention with the divine purpose are much more numerous than those that take a life.

The commitment to caring

Undoubtedly a tension exists between the health-care ethos of preserving life and the principle of respect for autonomy. It can be argued that to ask doctors and nurses to assist people to die runs counter to their basic commitment to help patients to live well. Certainly it would render them liable to prosecution in doubtful cases. It could, potentially, disturb the relationship which exists between them and their patients. Some would even argue that not having the right to help a person to die makes doctors strive ever harder to improve care for the terminally ill. This seems to suggest, however, that without such sanctions doctors would go in for widespread slaughter rather than working assiduously to ease the suffering of those they have in their care.

The slippery slope

The argument of the slippery slope is often used to answer the question of treating or not treating. It is suggested that once doctors and nurses are allowed to assist terminally ill people to die, the floodgates will be opened to a full extermination programme. In reality, decisions are made every day about whether it is appropriate to treat specific patients or not, and these decisions have been made for years. It would seem strange to single certain decisions out from the general continuum of care and suggest that these rather than the others lead to a degeneration of medical morals and standards.

Brutalizing effect

It is also sometimes argued that taking part in actions to hasten or allow death will have a brutalizing effect on doctors and nurses. Conscience plays a part here, as well as the influence of training and education. On a natural, intuitive, level alone we resist the idea of killing those we are trying to help. Equally, to stand by and witness the agony of someone dying in extreme pain can have a profound effect on carers. It raises the old question: if you saw someone slowly burning to death trapped in an upturned lorry would you shoot him to put him out of his misery when either alternative will result in certain death? It is hard to believe that compassionately assisting someone to end their suffering could be more brutalizing than standing by while an individual dies in torment.

Mistaken diagnosis

The statistics relating to the correlation between certified causes of death and causes found at postmortem are alarming indeed (Leadbetter and Knight 1993).

Anyone who has worked in intensive care units will know that some patients die in spite of our confidence in their ability to survive, and others survive when all our intuition, knowledge and experience tells us that they should not. These facts do indeed impinge on the debate. Can we really be sure of our diagnosis before we take such an irrevocable step?

Impaired judgement

An argument can be made around the possibility that the judgement of the patient may well be impaired at the time he decides to end his life. Indeed, it is well recognized that proximity to the diagnosis, mental state and circumstances produce varying reactions to the prospect of impending death. In my own work in the field of HIV/AIDS, I heard repeatedly that, faced with a new diagnosis of an incurable illness many patients contemplated suicide or euthanasia. However, as the weight of the diagnosis lifted and the prognosis extended in their experience, these young people fought the episodes of opportunistic infection with vigour, and some indeed fought death itself in the last stages of the disease with an amazing tenacity – one youth, for example, experienced Cheyne–Stokes respiration for 3 weeks before he finally died.

From this resum, of the main arguments it will be apparent that it is not a matter of listing the pros and cons, weighing them in the balance and deciding which is the most persuasive argument; rather it is careful scrutiny of the issues in each case which is needed. Facts, experience, judgement, values, beliefs, compassion and respect all enter into the equation before we arrive at a solution. We move on, then, to consider three scenarios which bring the issues into the real world as nurses know it. Examples are legion; these are merely illustrative. The full range of issues will not be examined. The cases are intended merely to demonstrate the complexity of the decision making, some of the principles we may apply, some of the lessons we may learn from history, and to give us some insight into our own attitudes, beliefs and values.

NURSING DILEMMAS

Resuscitation

Mr T. is a 56-year-old man brought unconscious into an accident and emergency (A&E) department. When he was picked up by the ambulance 7 miles away he was breathing spontaneously and his heart rate was faint and irregular. He appeared to be alone, and had no form of identification or medical information on his person to guide diagnosis. Shortly after admission he suffered a cardiac arrest.

It is almost inevitable that in these circumstances a resuscitation team will commence cardiopulmonary resuscitation. They have 3 minutes to act and no time to sit back considering objective data. There is a reflex response, the priority being to promote cardiac output and adequate ventilation; questions come later. Many know, all too painfully, the heavy consequences of their actions at times: the attempted suicide who ends up permanently brain damaged; the terminally ill patient who is brought back to life only to suffer more weeks of pain.

There are, of course, obvious advantages to starting life-sustaining measures. To begin with it buys time: time for mature reflection, for weighing up the burdens and benefits and for considering each aspect of the case calmly, with the available information more fully understood. It also allows proper consideration of the wishes and opinions of all the interested parties, both relatives and health workers.

Within most of us there is a degree of unwillingness to accept defeat. The number of attempts at resuscitation which go on long after intact survival is possible bear witness to this fact. In these days of audit we have to concern ourselves with departmental statistics. It is difficult, sometimes, to feel the weight of the quality of life arguments when we are looking at the number of our patients who have died. And rarely are these circumstances clearly defined and categorized. Logic and clinical judgement and compassion may well dictate different courses of action, and may lead us into different actions at various times in our lives and experiences.

Mr T.'s sister is found by the police living 40 miles away and she is brought in to visit him. She is his only surviving relative. As the days pass various tests show that Mr T. has suffered bilateral cerebral haemorrhages. He is totally paralysed and cannot speak. His state of semiconsciousness makes it impossible to ask what his wishes are, although his sister says she knows he would not want to continue in this half-alive state. He has always treasured his independence and dignity, but has never actually voiced what he would wish in the event of losing either or both.

Do we continue to treat this man vigorously? One alternative is to discontinue life-sustaining treatments, such as intravenous therapy and antibiotics for his chest infection, but many people find it difficult to withdraw having once started an aggressive course of treatment. Had we known at the outset that Mr T. faced this prognosis we might have been tempted to leave him alone in A&E. Now we have begun treatment, however, is it morally acceptable to change our minds and consign him to non-treatment? We know more about his circumstances and his prognosis. How can we decide?

The Institute of Medical Ethics (IME) Working Party (1990) has defined six constraints which ought to be considered. How do these apply to Mr T.?

- Respect for patient autonomy: We cannot ascertain what Mr T.'s wishes are and he is unable to communicate with us. He has left no advance directive.
- Duty to do no harm: Burdens must be carefully balanced against benefits. To continue to treat Mr T. is to sustain his life and keep a brother alive for his

only relative. This is at the expense of his loss of dignity and independence. We are reasonably confident that his quality of life will never improve.

● Justice and fair distribution of resources: Can we justify permitting Mr T. to become an appreciable drain on health service resources for the rest of his life? He will never again contribute anything tangible to society. It is difficult to see what he can contribute to his family and friends. On the other hand, what of the value of caring without hope of reward?

● Ruling out of alternatives: All potential avenues to relieve those things which encourage a person to end his life must be explored. Mental anguish, particularly, may be the result of pressures other than the illness itself. We cannot know what Mr T.'s mental state is because he cannot communicate it. It is essential that we do not assume that the way we think he must feel is actually how he feels. In this case even his nearest relative is only surmising.

● Necessity for collaboration: Working together as a team requires sensitivity, hearing all perspectives and understanding the effect of this experience on all those involved. A young nurse who has never seen such an ill person before and never watched someone die will probably experience this case quite differently from the older staff nurse whose mother suffered a cerebrovascular accident 4 years ago and lay in an unresponsive state for 6 months before she died.

● Respect for conscientious objection: Where any member of staff has a strong objection to participating in events which may hasten death, they should be given every opportunity to express their view. If, however, the consensus view is that Mr T. should be allowed to die peacefully and without further treatment, then the conscientious objector must be allowed to withdraw from the case.

The consensus decision is that in the event of collapse Mr T. will not be resuscitated. Inherent in this decision is the view that Mr T.'s life is not worth living and that death is a preferable state. Of course, it is hard for someone else to decide what amounts to a demonstrably awful existence and it very much depends on one's perspective. Many of us have repeatedly witnessed cases where terminally ill patients have fought to live long enough to experience some big event in their lives, and afterwards have given up the struggle.

Quality of life issues raise many questions. To put our present dilemma with Mr T. into this frame of reference, consider this quote from the Linacre Centre Working Party (1982):

'So the question being asked, implicitly, can be put thus: given his present 'quality of life', are the burdens of this (expensive or time-consuming or painful or disfiguring or undignified...) medical treatment worth enduring, in view of a) the probable 'quality of his life' while undergoing it and b) the probable 'quality of his life' if and when the treatment is completed.'

The use of quality of life as a criterion for decision-making about forgoing life-sustaining treatments has been heavily criticized: it smacks of discriminating against the disabled and the handicapped. But to leave it out is to ignore the practical consequences as they will be experienced by the patient and his family. This is not to say that all individuals will react in the same way to the possible impact of catastrophic impairment. However, if quality of life is not considered, it seems to imply that modern technology must be applied indiscriminately in all cases. Doctors and nurses become technicians rather than vulnerable individuals weighing up delicate medical, legal, emotional and ethical considerations.

Perhaps the real distinction relates to the focus of the decision-making. If we are considering the wisdom of a certain form of treatment, quality of life is part of the background informing that decision. On the other hand, if quality of life judgements are the focus, they become the basis and criteria for the selection of treatment, and potentially the rationale for a form of management which results in death.

Jennett (1982) has advocated a simpler list of questions to ask which nicely encapsulates the medical and the humane. He suggested that we ask whether treating the patient is likely to be unnecessary, unsuccessful, unwise, unsafe and/or unkind. In relation to Mr T. we can all make our own judgements on these bases. Your assessment might well differ in some degree from mine, but part of being accountable is addressing these issues for ourselves and making sure our practice is defensible in every way. The very richness of our diversity should ensure that the best interests of Mr T. and his sister are served.

To feed or not to feed

Sandra M. is a 24-year-old mother. Two years ago she was pushing her younger daughter in her pram under 40 feet of scaffolding when a girder smashed through the structure and fell on to her head and shoulders. She suffered appalling crush injuries and her baby daughter was killed outright. Sandra never regained consciousness, but a year ago was diagnosed as being in a persistent vegetative state. She lies now in a catatonic state, unaware of anyone or anything, breathing spontaneously but kept alive by means of a gastrostomy tube. Her husband visits her daily, occasionally bringing her little girl who is now 4½ years old. Sandra's parents also come to see her monthly, travelling 400 miles from their home expressly to do so. Both her parents and her husband have asked if she should be allowed to die.

Many of the issues we considered in relation to Mr T. apply here too, but there is an additional dilemma. The question being raised is: is it morally and legally permissible to stop feeding this patient? We have already seen the consternation caused by the suggestion that feeding be withdrawn from Tony Bland, lying similarly vegetatively. What is it that makes this decision so fraught with legal and moral peril?

Essentially this dilemma hinges around whether or not artificial feeding constitutes medical treatment. Legal experts have considered that:

'...artificial feeding inevitably requires some medical expertise and is, therefore, rightly considered part of selective medical treatment; the provision of food and water by normal means is the most elementary form of care owed to those who are helpless; how that should be provided is a matter of skilled nursing care' (Mason and McCall Smith 1991).

This statement underlines the unique role of nursing in the management of such patients and the necessity for the nursing profession to address their account-ability squarely rather than hide behind the doctor's larger responsibility.

There is a general consensus that in such cases feeding is a form of medical treatment. This was the conclusion of a panel of doctors, nurses and other professionals in the IME (IME Working Party 1991). In the United States, Justice Schreiber explicitly held that:

'...artificial feeding by means of a nasogastric tube...can be seen as equiv-alent to artificial breathing by means of a respirator. Both prolong life through mechanical means when the body is no longer able to perform a vital bodily function on its own' (Re Claire C. Conroy 1985).

The BMA has gone so far as to bring the quality of life into the argument:

'...feeding/gastrostomy tubes for nutrition and hydration are medical treat-ments and are warranted only when they make possible a decent life in which the patient can reasonably be thought to have continued interest' (BMA 1988).

Even the Roman Catholic stance, which traditionally is unequivocal on sanctity of life questions, has been that 'to persist in indiscriminately using such gestures [as artificial feeding regimens] can convey stupidity and cruelty, not compas-sion and love' (BMA 1992).

Why then the dilemma? It is often argued that giving food and fluid is a mark of continuing care and deference to the humanity of the patient. But the symbol-ism of these actions must not be allowed to eclipse their purpose. Although normally they equate to sustaining life, in some cases, such as persistent vegeta-tive state, they do not benefit patients since such patients feel nothing – they do not experience hunger and thirst. Thus in Sandra's case this issue is not really relevant. Even here medical and lay opinions can cause tensions. There are parents and families of patients in a persistent vegetative state who interpret reflex activity as cognitive response: a movement of the eyes or of a finger is interpreted as the patient communicating. They cannot believe or perhaps accept that their loved one is beyond their reach. If staff convey their experience to Sandra's husband or parents, doubts may well be put into minds once sure of what they wanted. A very natural need to hope, and not to destroy the hope of others, may well eclipse rational argument and medical experience. Subsequent decisions may be more reflective of the comfort of the carers than of the patient, and must be recognized as such.

Potential conflict may also occur between the professionals, or between the health-care staff and the family. Miles (1987) observed that doctors tend to equate feeding with a medical treatment to achieve physiological ends, whereas families see it as an 'act of community'. It is important to recognize these different meanings. It has been clearly established that withdrawing artificial feeding does not lead to distressing signs and symptoms if appropriate nursing care is given (Schmitz and O'Brien 1986; Cranford 1988). Here, again, the vital role of nursing is highlighted. On a purely practical level it is nurses who must ensure good mouth care in order to prevent unpleasant symptoms developing, and who perhaps help the family to realize the true position, possibly even encouraging them to participate in these last acts of caring. Nurses have, however, been found to fear that withholding hydration will cause discomfort or distress (Davidson *et al.* 1990), and something of this general belief may well influence the staff closely involved with Sandra as long as she is seen as a human being. Her insentient state is difficult to comprehend fully, and niggling doubts about the paucity of information from the patient's point of view may linger and cloud otherwise rational thinking.

A number of cases relating to the withdrawal of feeding have made legal history (Steinbrook and Lo 1988), but an emerging consensus has been seen. The patient's wishes should be taken as the focus of discussion: competent patients have a right to refuse feeding if they assess the burdens as far outweighing the benefits; where a person is incompetent, feeding may be stopped in accordance with previously expressed wishes. This is not to say that there is unanimous agreement on these matters, or that the ethical position is now clear. There is still considerable debate and many unresolved issues remain.

In Sandra's case she had never discussed such matters with her relatives so it is impossible to know what her wishes might have been. She is not competent to refuse feeding or to weigh up the burdens and benefits of further treatment. Some form of substituted judgement has to be made. But whose interests are we considering? As far as Sandra is concerned she feels no pain and is not troubled by her vegetative state, so we cannot suggest that it is in her best interests to be dead – it does not matter to her either way. For her husband and parents there is more at stake. They are suffering enormously from seeing the person they love in a pitiful state, unable to be reached in any meaningful way. They might well feel that mourning her death is to be preferred to the daily corrosive sorrow of witnessing her tragic survival. On the other hand, they may be reluctant to face the final parting, or to contemplate the potential guilt and pain from making a decision for her dying. Sandra's daughter is too young to have her opinion taken very seriously. Who is to say how she will react to the outcome in years to come, or how this present experience of being unable to communicate with her mother will have affected her? And how will such a decision affect the community this hospital serves? Will they be perceived as compassionate or will they face hostility as if they were executioners, lightly dispensing with human life?

The feelings and values of the staff are also relevant. Over 2 years they will have established a relationship with this family. They too suffer feelings of anger, frustration and sorrow. For each one of them the dividing line between the positive and the negative aspects of Sandra's continued existence may be at a different place along the continuum. Whose responsibility is it actually to remove or not replace her feeding tube? Who will keep vigil at her bedside as she dies? As we can readily understand, it is a matter of life and death how professionals reason in these cases. Thus, it is imperative that all individuals examine their ethical reasoning as a matter of some urgency.

The incompetent patient

Timothy W. is a 23-week-gestation infant weighing just 430 kg. His parents are in their late 30s and have been trying to have a family for 15 years. Although his Apgar scores were initially good, Timothy's condition rapidly deteriorated and he is now on full ventilation, with grade 4 ventricular haemorrhages and a poor prognosis. His parents are aware of the implications for his future were he to survive. Severe impairment is a virtual certainty. They also know that any aggressive management carries a burden of pain and distress for their baby. They are asked to decide whether they wish heroic measures to be continued or whether they wish all treatment to be discontinued and little Timothy allowed to die cradled in their arms for his last few hours of life.

Perhaps nowhere is the problem of the 'incompetent to decide' patient raised more acutely than in the case of neonates, for when it comes to infants whose lives have only just begun, the debate becomes heavily overladen with emotion. Unlike most other categories of such seriously ill people, they have no history to guide us. We cannot know their wishes or their stamina or their beliefs, nor with any certainty what their potential is nor how much of it they will realize. Even their religious affiliation is inferred by virtue of their parentage, although this can have a major effect on the choices available.

Nor is past precedent much of a guide. Such conflicting accounts as severely handicapped adults or their carers have given show us that what is a demonstrably awful existence to one is not so to another; and what can seem intolerable in anticipation can turn out to be an intolerable burden indeed, or it may become, in retrospect, a refining experience bringing unexpected blessings. No one can know for sure which way it may go.

It is only rarely that such a decision must be made on the spot. Most neonatologists appear to subscribe to the view that initial active resuscitation is appropriate. It allows a considered decision to be made on accumulating evidence about whether to continue to treat or not. Nevertheless, a minority, recognizing the pain and awfulness of treatment, prefer to take a rapid decision and simply do not begin to treat an infant with a very poor prognosis (Utley 1992).

The legal issues have been contested over many years with landmark cases, and have largely been decided on a case-by-case basis. Different agents debating the wisdom of treating infants in specific ways have exposed the 'minefield' that neonatal care presents. The very public trial of Dr Arthur, who prescribed lethal doses of dihydrocodeine for a child with Down's syndrome, brought matters very much into the public domain (Brahams 1981). The cases of Baby Alexandra, also with Down's syndrome, but with an accompanying intestinal obstruction (Re B. 1981), and Baby J. born at 27 weeks' gestation, who subsequently developed severe brain damage (Re J. 1990), preoccupied various courts for lengthy periods of time. Almost inevitably there is a range of people who might well feel they can best offer a substituted judgement. Tensions will arise.

As we have seen in the cases of Mr T. and Sandra, quality of life issues are relevant but give rise to ambiguity and tension. As long ago as 1973, Duff and Campbell raised the issue of quality of life in relation to treating neonates, breaking the 'public and professional silence on a major social taboo'. The question had become not 'can' but 'should' it be done? They observed that the issues, no matter how much we might resist them, were not to be brushed aside:

'...the awesome finality of these decisions, combined with a potential for error in prognosis, made the choice agonizing for families and health professionals. Nevertheless, the issue has to be faced, for not to decide is an arbitrary and potentially devastating decision of default' (Duff and Campbell 1973).

Neonatal care, perhaps more than most other medical specialties, highlights the three obligations that doctors and nurses must consider: to the patient, to the family and to society. Making decisions in the highly charged atmosphere of a neonatal intensive care unit is something which affects the participants deeply and reaches into their inner beliefs and values – about themselves and about life and society, as well as about the family in question. It can be very threatening. Not all professionals are prepared to challenge their own feelings about such fundamental matters and may avoid situations where they are required to do so. In the case of Timothy, issues relating to death itself are confounded and complicated by those of society's and individuals' reactions to the severely handicapped, to infertility, to the allocation of scarce resources, and to family love and contact.

Perhaps not surprisingly, given their approach to euthanasia, doctors in The Netherlands have addressed these issues head-on. The Dutch Society of Paediatrics has recently reported the conclusions of its deliberations in a report, *To Do or Not to Do? Boundaries for Medical Action in Neonatology*. A distinction is made between medical action which has no chance of success (such as where an infant will certainly die in a short space of time) and action which has the potential to succeed but is unethical because it is pointless (such as those infants with a prognosis so bad that their lives would be unbearable). An unlivable life needs some kind of definition, and five criteria have been laid down. It is decided upon with reference to i) the ability to communicate verbally and non-verbally with others; ii) the ability to look after oneself; iii) the degree of dependence on medical support; iv) the degree of suffering both present and future; and v) life expectancy (Hellema 1992). However, if we consider Timothy's life against these criteria we can see the potential ambiguity and the range of unknowns which put obstacles in the path of decision making, even with such guidelines. It cannot be said with any certainty just how much he will be able to communicate at this stage. These things emerge slowly. His degree of independence will be determined by factors in addition to his medical condition; his parents' ability and support, and his own stamina and approach to life, will be germane to this issue; all these factors are as yet unknown. Almost certainly he will need ongoing medical support, but so do patients on kidney dialysis and no-one seems to be suggesting that they should simply be left to die.

Assessing the degree of suffering, both present and future, is equally problematical. While Timothy is a tiny infant housed in an incubator his impairments are scarcely apparent. He may be cuddled and touched and admired in much the same way as any intact child of his age and size. At 1 year his differences will be more noticeable, but he can still be lovable and his parents may derive pleasure from contact with his living frame. As he grows and his differences become more apparent and his behaviour less socially acceptable, his demands on both physical and mental strength will certainly increase. Who can possibly predict whether his parents will still feel that the benefits of his continued existence outweigh the burdens in years to come? His life expectancy may be predicted on the basis of statistics, but many and graphic are the accounts of those who have defied the statistics and it is extremely difficult for those intimately wrapped up in the fate of a baby to assess the relative risks dispassionately.

Even such a superficial consideration of the criteria shows how great is the task of deciding. The professionals involved will need patience, tact and strength to guide parents through such an agonizing experience to a final choice. They must each be aware of the issues and their own stance in relation to them if they are to conduct themselves in a way that takes full account of the awesome responsibility of their task.

THE REALITY

One point needs to be emphasized at this juncture: deciding not to treat does not mean abandonment, or withdrawing care; rather, it should involve an increased commitment to the patient and the family, as Campbell (1992) has eloquently argued. Nursing's contribution here is vital. As well as their important role in decision making, the nurses' constant attendance, sharing of the experience, being with and listening to the family, forms a large part of the support such individuals inevitably need.

There is, however, sometimes a difference between what we know we ought to do to care and what we actually do. To begin with, our own prejudices and judgements can get in the way. There are, too, limits to our mental and emotional stamina. The higher our own concept of the ethical ideal of caring, the greater the potential for a shortfall. Competing demands, differences between what we think the patient wants and what the relatives think the patient wants, tensions with colleagues, and sometimes outright conflict and a sense of guilt, can all confound and plague us. Sometimes a simple need to protect ourselves can lead us to choose to offer a service rather than really care (Brown *et al.* 1992).

Strength lies in team effort. No one individual should be required to shoulder the entire burden of such an awesome decision. Reasonable people may legitimately hold different views about the moral acceptability of the management of a case where it is based on their evaluation of the burdens and benefits to the individual, the family or society. The different ways by which people ethically reason (Uden *et al.* 1992); differing values, motivations and expectations (Grundstein-Amado 1992); and each discipline's perceptions of the other (Uden *et al.* 1992) may well contribute to individuals holding varying opinions about any given case. If there were a 'right' answer, dilemmas would not occur with such worrying frequency. Disagreement, however, need not be a negative experience degenerating into destructive conflict; rather, it can be a strength, safeguarding patients' welfare. It is the way in which disagreements are handled that makes the difference.

Even where careful and respectful communication and collaboration are practised, there will be unhappiness and failures to resolve difficult situations. Simply by virtue of the powerful feelings and beliefs being compromised, there will be trauma to certain individuals. It is important not to shy away from reflecting on these decisions after the event. The very complexity and lack of absolutes makes it almost inevitable that doubts will remain in some cases. Using these constructively can only refine our judgement and our caring skills.

CONCLUSION

Involving all interested parties in these grave decisions is not yet universally practised. An international survey of practitioners in intensive care showed that, while the majority did discuss matters with the families, only 7% involved the patient in the decision as to whether or not they were for resuscitation. Vincent (1990) concluded that these questions remain very difficult to ask. Perhaps, more worryingly, only about half involved the nurses and other intensive care unit staff. For nurses to ensure that they are actively involved in these decision-making processes is one step that might effect healthy change.

Fostering an adaptable and flexible approach is an essential prerequisite. Over 1000 nurses responded to a survey by the *Nursing Times* in 1988. They showed clearly that in their perception the edges of these issues are blurred. The widely differing responses indicate that each case needs to be considered individually, and that blanket dictates are inappropriate. Clearly, if nurses are to contribute wisely, they need to have thought through the issues carefully. To a degree the underlying ethical principles can be taught, but it is no use coming out of a course understanding the meaning of the principles of beneficence or non-maleficence or autonomy if these things are not applied to the actual business of nursing real live patients. We return to our initial thesis that these matters have to be firmly rooted in the day-to-day situations which confront nurses in their practice.

An element of risk is inherent in the practice of responsible nursing. However, nurses must know their own ethical position and decide for themselves the boundaries of their personal and professional responsibilities. Exercising this awareness in terms of specific cases will hone their skills in decision-making and, used appropriately, will healthily underpin their stance with facts and sound information.

Maybe, however, we need more than simply education about ethical and moral reasoning more than exercises in assertiveness. It is possible that nurses, like society at large, need to rethink their attitude to death itself. Survival can be a greater disaster than death. Life at any price is no longer acceptable. 'For nurses, the experience of truly and personally caring for a patient affirms the fullest potential in their professional practice' (Olsen 1992), and perhaps nowhere is this caring more essentially the nub of the quality of life for a patient than in his last hours. It is not always possible to cure; it should always be possible to care enough to offer comfort and compassion. Such caring will exact a price, as was seen in the case of the nurses who cared for the Bland family through all the vicissitudes of their ordeal (Alderman 1993). A degree of suffering is, however, the price we pay for caring.

Some people have expressed suspicion of any form of expertise when it comes to these momentous life and death decisions. They worry about who will monitor the experts (Utley 1992). Having patrolled the corridors of medicine and nursing for many years, it is my considered view that the agony which each of these decisions engenders is itself the safeguard we need in order to protect nursing and medicine from sliding down the 'slippery slope'. These decisions are not made in a vacuum. The pain and individual heart searching; the informed and respectful challenging of each other; and the process of sifting the relevant factors in order to reach a decision guided by the 'best interests' argument, will be more effective than any outside policing. This is not to say that these matters should not be open to public scrutiny. Such examination should simply show that those who are most closely involved are behaving in a moral and compassionate way by taking account of the circumstances and family wishes in each individual case, and that professional accountability is taken seriously.

If, then, we are to do justice to the breadth and depth of nursing in all its complexity and uniqueness, we owe it to the profession, as well as to ourselves individually, to address these issues squarely. We each need to test our opinions and values, measure our limits and analyse our sticking points. And we need to do all this as far as possible before these matters challenge each one of us profoundly and personally. After all, we do not see best when our eyes are full of tears.

PART FIVE:

Research and Education

13

Accountability in nursing research

Alison J. Tierney

INTRODUCTION

Accountability has come to be regarded as a key concept for nursing in its pursuit of the kind of autonomy which is enjoyed by other professions, notably medicine. Concern with the notion of accountability has been most obvious in connection with interests in primary nursing and, more recently, the named nurse concept. Individual accountability is the cornerstone of these ideas which, in the United Kingdom at least, are quite novel. They certainly represent a radical departure from traditional forms of nursing within the old-style hierarchical structure, in which military principles and then line management inculcated unquestioning obedience rather than any sense of personal responsibility and individual accountability for professional practice.

Most of the discussion and the literature relating to accountability in nursing has centred on nursing practice. Interestingly, the matter of accountability in the field of nursing research has not been much written about and yet, as this chapter hopefully will demonstrate, it impinges on the everyday work of the nurse researcher and each stage of the research process.

RESEARCH AS A RESPONSIBILITY OF AN ACCOUNTABLE PROFESSION

It is now generally acknowledged that, if nurses are to be truly accountable for their practice in a professional sense, then they must accept responsibility, both individually and collectively, for advancing the knowledge base of nursing. For a very long time the nursing profession seemed content with practice and organizational approaches which were based on tradition and routine rather than research. It was therefore a significant departure for the profession when the Briggs Committee, reporting on its wide-ranging review of British nursing as it entered the 1970s, recommended that 'nursing should become a research-based profession' and declared that 'a sense of the need for research should become a part of the mental equipment of every practising nurse' (HMSO 1972).

At that time, the amount of research activity in nursing was very limited indeed. Only a few nurses had accumulated research experience and fewer still had undergone formal research training. Research posts, or even posts with attached research responsibilities, were rare. The basic nursing curriculum paid scant attention to research and, indeed, students could reach the end of their training without ever having been introduced to research. Nurses in practice were either unconcerned with research or hostile to the introduction of an apparently unnecessary 'academic' approach in a practical profession.

Times have changed. Worldwide, nursing is an increasingly research-aware and research-active profession. The amount of research being undertaken has grown steadily over the past 20 years, as is evident in nursing's burgeoning literature, including a healthy amount of research material in the so-called popular press. Research is no longer seen as the prerogative of 'academic nursing', but as both a right and a responsibility in all sections of the profession.

Nursing's achievements in the field of research over a comparatively short timespan, and with relatively limited resources, are impressive. But it is equally important for the profession to acknowledge that its research capability remains weak, and that a clear strategy for future development is essential. In this respect, the *Strategy for Research in Nursing, Midwifery and Health Visiting*, which was formulated by a task force on behalf of the Department of Health (DoH 1993b), with counterparts in the other United Kingdom countries, represents an important step forward for the profession.

The Strategy underlines the growing importance of research in nursing as a necessary base for practice and, overall, for professional accountability in this era of health service reform, with its emphasis on measurable outcomes and cost-effectiveness. The need for research evidence which demonstrates cost-effectiveness is particularly important in relation to nursing because of its use of such a sizeable element of the overall health service budget.

Rightly, the task force drew attention to the lack of such evidence and the generally limited impact of past research in nursing. It also reminded individual nurses, as accountable practitioners, of their key responsibility as research users. For the producers of research, the task force points out the serious limitations of a continuing proliferation of small-scale inconsequential studies. Recognition of the need for a shift to stronger 'science' in nursing research is implicit in the definition of research adopted by the task force:

'...rigorous and systematic enquiry, conducted on a scale and using methods commensurate with the issue to be investigated, and designed to lead to generalizable contributions to knowledge.'

It is from research findings that have a potential for generalization that a robust knowledge base for nursing will be accumulated most efficiently, allowing practice and policy to be based firmly on research.

The development of a coherent and comprehensive strategy for nursing research in the United Kingdom is timely. Throughout the health service there is a growing recognition of the necessity and value of research. The need for research to become an integral part of strategic health service planning, day-to-day decision-making and ongoing evaluation is the basic premise of the *Research and Development Strategy* which has been formulated by the Government for the health service as a whole (DoH 1991b; SOHHD 1993). The strategy for nursing research is separate from, but congruent with, this overall strategy.

The *Research and Development Strategy* emphasizes the need for research priorities to relate more closely to the current priorities of the health service itself, so that research contributes directly to 'health gain' and to improvements in standards, efficiency and effectiveness of health care. It is recognized that, in order to achieve this, there must be closer cooperation than in the past between researchers of different disciplines, as well as between the research community as a whole and health service managers and practitioners. There is the need too, it is argued, for stronger accountability for the public funds put into research and development activities within the health service. Thus, research is now being seen, in nursing as in the health service at large, as a responsibility of all accountable professionals and any publicly accountable organization.

ACCOUNTABILITY IN NURSING RESEARCH

Having set the context in terms of research as a responsibility of an accountable profession, and the use of research as a responsibility of each individual member of that profession as an accountable practitioner, attention turns now to the subject of accountability in nursing research. This chapter concentrates on an exploration of the exercise of personal accountability by nurses whose sole or primary occupation is research. Most of what is said, however, will have relevance for any nurse who, despite having another primary professional function, is directly or indirectly involved in research.

Nurse researchers as nurses – a personal angle

Are nurse researchers nurses or researchers first? Although a career researcher working in a university environment, I still regard myself first and foremost as a nurse by profession. In much the same way, other academics who have established a career in medical or health services research may still identify themselves as epidemiologists, sociologists or health economists.

As a nurse, and having maintained active registration with the UKCC (the United Kingdom Central Council for Nursing, Midwifery and Health Visiting), I therefore regard the UKCC *Code of Professional Conduct* as being as applicable to me as to any nurse. The code (UKCC 1992a) aims to 'safeguard and promote the interests of individual patients and clients; serve the interests of society; justify public trust and confidence; and uphold and enhance the good standing and reputation of the professions'. All of these aims are as pertinent to nursing research as to any other area of professional nursing.

The code goes on to say that 'as a registered nurse, midwife or health visitor, you are personally accountable for your practice'. Again, this is as applicable to a nurse researcher as to any nurse. Although the ensuing specifications in the code regarding the exercise of professional accountability were apparently written with practising nurses in mind, each of the 16 'rules' has direct or indirect relevance for nurse researchers. Indeed, many seem particularly pertinent: for example, those that refer to the primacy of patients' interests and wellbeing (1); the requirement of necessary knowledge and competence (4); the avoidance of abuse of a nurse's privileged relationship with patients (9); the legal and moral rules on confidentiality of information (10); the sharing of knowledge (14); and the need to protect professional judgement from the influence of commercial or other considerations (16).

Although these clauses will not be examined systematically, many of the implicit issues will be raised in the course of this chapter. The UKCC Code of Professional Conduct provides a relevant and very useful backdrop to an exploration of personal accountability in the sphere of nursing research.

Defining accountability

Interestingly, the UKCC code does not make explicit the underlying definition of accountability. Having reached this stage of the book, you will have been exposed to a variety of definitions and perspectives and, of course, it is necessary for each contributor to make clear how accountability is being defined. My own understanding derives from the simple definition in my regular dictionary (*The Oxford Reference Dictionary*). There, 'accountable' is defined as 'having to account (for one's actions)'; 'to account for' as 'to give a reckoning of'; and 'an account' as 'a description, a report'.

By these definitions, accountability is a familiar notion to a researcher. Indeed, perhaps in more detail than those working in other fields of practice, researchers are required to provide a full and formal written account of their work – both in advance (i.e. the research protocol) and on completion (the research report). In the technical sense, too, there is an accounting component in both of these written documents, since the researcher initially costs the project when drawing up a research budget and, at the end, a report on actual expenditure will be required.

The importance of accountability in research

By this simple analysis it is clear that accountability is an important, integral aspect of research. It seems strange, then, that it has been so neglected in the literature. Perhaps accountability in research is taken so much for granted, and its exercise in practice regarded as so straightforward, that the need for analysis and debate has not been felt.

This lack of attention is not peculiar to nursing. The issue of accountability in research in any field rarely seems to be a routine matter of public or professional debate. Questions of accountability in research really only come to the fore when a case of academic fraud or financial indiscretion in the use of research funds is exposed. What these cases tend to reveal is the high degree of autonomy that researchers enjoy, and the extent to which their work is (or can be) conducted in privacy – even secrecy – and how rare it is for researchers to be called publicly to account for the conduct and results of their research.

The other side of this coin, of course, is that researchers must accept a high degree of personal responsibility for the quality and integrity of their work, and for the proper use of research funds. With personal responsibility comes individual accountability. The researcher's final account (i.e. the research report) will be scrutinized by the funding body and then, in published form, the account will become available for open critical appraisal by experts and peers. If a researcher's account is found wanting, at best further grants will be hard or impossible to obtain, and at worst there will be no further career prospects in research. In scandalous cases there may even be public disgrace.

In comparison with 'high science', the world of nursing research has been concerned with modest amounts of money, and with research issues which are rarely seen as having huge importance. There has been no great public or professional interest in the standards or regulation of nursing research. To my knowledge, no nurse has been struck off the register for improprieties in the conduct of research. Except for large-scale projects, or programmes which are government-funded, the outputs of research in nursing are seldom subjected to the degree of scrutiny and criticism that is commonplace in other disciplines.

Changing times?

Times are changing. Assume that the strategic plans to strengthen research in nursing and to integrate it more closely with increased research and development activity in the health service as a whole are implemented. If this happens, then there will be more money invested in nursing research and, as a consequence, it will become subjected to more external and stringent scrutiny than in the past. Inevitably there will be expectations of higher standards and greater accountability. The considerable degree of autonomy that nurse researchers have been able to enjoy may be challenged. Accountability is likely to become less a matter of personal integrity and more a matter of public interest and formal regulation. This will happen as the organizations in which nurse researchers work (i.e. the health service and the universities) are themselves called to account in greater detail for their use of money and manpower in the pursuit of research.

TO WHOM ARE NURSE RESEARCHERS ACCOUNTABLE?

By definition, accountability is to another party or parties, including those in positions of authority, but interestingly also to those who are in positions of equality and dependence. Whereas accountability to those in positions of authority arises from the notion of 'dueness', the idea of 'duty' is connected with accountability to those in equal or dependent positions. Both of these terms – dueness and duty – are linked (for example in *Roget's Thesaurus*) with the concept of accountability, and both apply in the context of research.

In the field of practice, nurses are accountable to their clients, the profession, their manager and their employing organization, as well as to themselves, according to Evans (1993). The same sort of mix applies in the field of research. Accountability in the case of nurse researchers will be examined in relation to the sponsor (i.e. the grant-giving body); research ethics committees (the main purpose of which is to protect the public); research participants; those who control research access (the 'gatekeepers'); co-researchers; the profession (i.e. the research consumers); and, finally, the wider public.

Accountability to the sponsor

For any researcher, probably the most formal line of accountability is to the sponsor – i.e. the grant-giving body. Indeed, ensuring that a research project is adequately financed from the outset is a prime responsibility of an accountable researcher. This principle applies irrespective of the size of a project. All research costs money. There are always labour costs and, even in the most modest of projects, there will be at least some material costs as well. Gone are the days when health service staff might have managed to conduct a research survey 'for free' by cajoling the ward secretary into typing the questionnaire and donating the envelopes, and then putting these out through the hospital mail. Even the smallest of research projects needs a budget and this in turn requires a sponsor.

Who are the sponsors?

Sponsorship for a nursing research study can be sought from a wide range of sources. Government funding is a major source of finance for studies in nursing and health care. In Scotland, research funding for such studies is disbursed through the Chief Scientist Office of the Scottish Office Home and Health Department in the form of grants for projects and mini-projects. Awards are made on the basis of peer review of research grant applications and committee agreement. Equivalent arrangements exist in the other health departments, and similarly well-defined grant-awarding systems are operated by the research councils, the most relevant to nursing being the Medical Research Council (MRC) and the Economic and Social Research Council (ESRC).

The NHS itself has a budget for research and, in the wake of the Research and Development Strategy, this has increased substantially. Staff working in the NHS, nurses included, can apply for these research funds through whatever mechanism exists in their own health region. It is possible, too, for research funds to be accessed even more locally – i.e. from available sources within a particular directly managed unit or trust. Beyond government and the NHS, funding for research in the field of health care is available from a host of charitable trusts as well as from the commercial sector, including pharmaceutical companies and other suppliers. There is no shortage of funds for nursing research: the challenge is for nurses to become more successful at accessing the funds which are available to the research community as a whole.

How is accountability to sponsors defined?

Irrespective of the source or amount of funding, all sponsors enter into some form of contractual relationship with the researcher. The researcher may be expected to be directly accountable to the sponsor, or the line of accountability may be through an intermediary, for example the head of department in the case of a nurse researcher based in a university, or a general manager or clinical director in the case of a nurse who is an NHS employee. These more senior members of the organization concerned may be appointed formally by the sponsor as the grant-holder and, in such cases, they are the people to whom the researcher is accountable on a day-to-day basis, and through them to the sponsor.

The contract will (or, at least, should) also specify the terms and conditions of the grant. The sponsor should make clear what the grant is supporting and when accounts are due, and in what form. In most cases, the usual expectation is for a final report to be submitted by a specified date but, in the case of some sponsors or in longer studies, interim reports might be required as well. A sponsor has every right, of course, to dictate the conditions of the grant. It is in the researcher's own interests to know exactly what is being expected and to accept the grant only if the sponsor's conditions are acceptable and manageable.

Particular care needs to be taken in this respect when research sponsorship is provided by a commercial organization. The UKCC Code of Professional Conduct (paragraph 16) warns nurses to 'ensure that your registration is not used in the promotion of commercial products or services, (to) declare any financial or other interests in relevant organizations providing such goods or services and ensure that your professional judgement is not influenced by any commercial considerations'. Thus, for example, special care would be required to maintain a totally objective stance in a research project on infant feeding which is funded by a manufacturer of artificial milk products, and freedom to publish the results (irrespective of the findings) should be established as the researcher's right at the outset. In relation to this kind of issue, the guidelines provided by the Royal College of Nursing (RCN 1993b) advise that 'researchers must make clear to sponsors, employers and colleagues that research does not necessarily guarantee solutions to problems, and should make explicit the limitations and likely benefits of the proposed research'.

Once agreed, the sponsor's conditions are set out in a letter or, in the case of larger grant-giving bodies, in a formal contract. The latter has been the custom, for example, in the case of a grant from the Chief Scientist Office (Scottish Office), the terms being set out in a document called Conditions of Grant. Before the grant is released this kind of document is usually required to be signed by all parties who will be held accountable by the sponsor for the satisfactory completion of the project and the agreed deployment of the funds.

Failure to comply with the conditions of grant during the course of the project could result in withdrawal of the sponsor's support. If there is failure to complete the work satisfactorily, or to deliver the agreed 'products', it is likely that the researcher(s) concerned would be deemed ineligible to apply for funds from that grant-giving body for future research.

Thus, a researcher's relationship with the sponsor, whether in a direct or indirect line of accountability, is a formal contractual relationship and, as such, it should be clearly defined and understood from the outset.

Accountability to research ethics committees

There is a similarly formal process of accountability in relation to research ethics committees. The undertaking of any nursing (or health-related) research project which involves human subjects, whether directly or indirectly, requires the prior approval of the appropriate research ethics committee/s. The role of these committees is to ensure that all research in the health-care field is ethically sound. In order to obtain ethical approval, the researcher submits the research protocol along with a statement of the ethical implications of the proposed study and a description of the procedures that will be followed to ensure that the undertaking will be ethically sound. The format of the submission and the way the committees work varies from place to place, and therefore details of the procedures in place locally must be obtained by contacting the health authority/board in whose area the research is to be conducted.

What is ethical research?

A short but helpful account of the ethical principles underpinning research is provided in the introduction to the booklet on *Ethics Related to Research in*

Nursing (RCN 1993b), which was formulated by the Research Advisory Group of the Royal College of Nursing. Beneficence (doing good to people) and non-maleficence (doing them no harm) are identified as two ethical principles of major importance in research. According to Thompson *et al.* (1994), 'in order to be ethical, nursing research must be based on prior assessment of risks and benefits of the research procedures' and they argue that a research project 'would not be justified when the risks outweigh the benefits'.

Assuming that the proposed research fulfils these fundamental conditions, other ethical principles of importance (as mentioned in the RCN booklet) include the principle of fidelity (trust), because research subjects entrust themselves to the researcher; the principle of justice (being fair), because research must not exploit people; the principle of autonomy (self-determination), which underpins the condition of voluntary informed consent; the principle of veracity (truth-telling), which is crucial in terms of the information given to patients as well as in the eventual reporting of the research; and, of course, the principle of confidentiality which, in research as in other spheres of professional practice, has legal as well as ethical dimensions.

Research can be designed from the outset to be ethically sound if steps are taken to address each of these principles in the course of developing a research proposal. There are, of course, some research topics and designs which have an inherently complex ethical dimension, and some client groups (for example children, the mentally ill, the frail elderly and the dying) pose particularly difficult moral dilemmas for the researcher. Somehow, these need to be resolved if the researcher is to be morally accountable, and indeed the concepts of ethics and accountability are inextricably linked.

Being 'morally accountable'

In a formal sense, the researcher's 'moral accountability' is to the research ethics committee. When the committee gives its ethical approval there is the expectation that the researcher will conduct the research exactly as planned, including adhering to any procedures designed specifically to safeguard ethical soundness. Occasionally ethics committees do engage in direct monitoring of the conduct of the approved research; sometimes they require periodic progress reports, but more often the ethical conduct of the research is entrusted to the researcher. Thus, moral accountability depends essentially on the personal integrity of the individual researcher.

Even for the most conscientious individual this can be taxing. Take, for example, a project in which frail elderly people are involved and, because of their recognized vulnerability, the ethics committee has been particularly demanding about the procedure to be used for ensuring informed voluntary consent.

First there is the task of deciding what information about the research must be given to the potential subjects, and how it should be presented. The information must be presented very clearly (whether verbally or in writing, or both) and it must be sufficient in detail but, for elderly people, not over-complicated, as this may cause confusion or unnecessary anxiety. Then there is the need to work out a practical procedure for imparting the information and obtaining the patient's consent, usually involving a formal signature.

In theory the procedure is simple enough, but in practice it can be less than straightforward. On initial approach, elderly patients may be wary of the whole idea of research or, in contrast, willing to submit unquestioningly to any request, especially one coming from a nurse. Should the former be subjected to persuasion and the latter encouraged to exercise caution? And what of the old person who is quite happy to sign the consent form but does not seem to have studied (or understood) the information? In any case, how does the researcher ever really know that the given consent is truly both informed and voluntary? Any researcher, quite naturally, feels under pressure to recruit the required number of subjects, and when the procedures which were approved by the ethics committee have been dutifully followed, there is every temptation to accept consent at face value and to set aside any niggling doubts about its authenticity.

Being morally accountable is a demanding aspect of research. Ethics committees have an important role to play in safeguarding the ethical soundness of research, but the maintenance of ethical standards is largely dependent on the discretion and integrity of the individual researcher.

Accountability to research participants

Whereas grant-giving bodies and research ethics committees are in positions of authority and have a degree of 'hold' over the researcher's exercise of account-ability, the subjects of research are in a relatively powerless position. Attention has been drawn already to the distinction between duty and dueness in account-ability. Acknowledgement of the dependence of research subjects is especially important in nursing and health services research. It is usually the case that research subjects are recruited while they are patients and, as such, occupying a position of dependence in the system (as distinct from a position of authority or equality). Patients may thus feel a sense of obligation to participate in the research.

Basic principles

The nurse researcher, as nurse, will safeguard the interests of patients if guided by the foremost principles of the UKCC Code of Conduct (paragraphs 1 and 2). These state that in the exercise of professional accountability the nurse must 'act always in such a manner as to promote and safeguard the interests and well-being of patients and clients'; and 'ensure that no action or omission on your part, or within your sphere of responsibility, is detrimental to the interests, condition or safety of patients and clients'. These basic principles are as pertinent to the work of a nurse researcher as to that of any practising nurse.

Further, the code (paragraph 9) points out the necessity to 'avoid any abuse of your privileged relationship with patients and clients and of the privileged access allowed to their person, property, residence or workplace'. This is an important principle, particularly for nurses who are engaged in 'on-the-job' research and are recruiting for research purposes those patients with whom they are already involved as practitioners. In such situations, clear delineation, for the patient, of the nurse's dual roles is imperative if abuse of the nurse's pre-existing privileged relationship and access is to be avoided.

A nurse researcher 'from outside', of course, does not have such a relationship. In my experience, however, patients do tend to accord a nurse researcher the kind of sympathy and willingness to oblige that they tend to give to nurses in general. There may be merit, therefore, in the researcher concealing their identity as a nurse, particularly if there is no reason in terms of the patient's interests why this should be declared.

Respecting autonomy

In exercising accountability to research participants, respect for their autonomy is a basic premise. The necessity for, and importance of, involving research subjects on the basis of informed voluntary consent has already been mentioned. On this subject, the RCN (1993b) spells out what is involved:

> 'Researchers are responsible for obtaining freely given and informed consent from each individual who is to be a subject of study or, in some other way, personally involved in the research. This requires that the researcher explain as fully as possible, and in terms meaningful to the subjects, the nature and purpose of the study, how and why they were selected and invited to take part, what is required of them and who is undertaking and financing the investigation. This information should be provided in written form at all times; the subject's consent, whether written or verbal, should be recorded.'

Further, the RCN guidelines draw attention to the fact that respect for the autonomy of research participants is an ongoing responsibility of the researcher:

> 'In seeking voluntary informed consent, the researcher must emphasize that the subjects have an absolute right to refuse to participate or to withdraw from the study at any time without their care being affected in any way. The rights of refusal and withdrawal must be totally respected by researchers.'

In exercising accountability in research, therefore, the matter of respect for the autonomy of participants is of paramount importance.

Fulfilling pledges of confidentiality

Another key issue that concerns accountability to research subjects is confidentiality. The UKCC Code of Professional Conduct (paragraph 10) makes clear that, in the exercise of professional accountability, the nurse must 'protect all confidential information concerning patients and clients obtained in the course of professional practice and make disclosures only with consent'. The RCN Ethical Guidelines for Nursing Research draw attention to the fact that 'researchers should be aware that personal health information, such as is held in medical records and nursing notes, is confidential and therefore permission and consent are required for its use in research'. Further, the guidelines point out that 'the nature of any promises of confidentiality or restriction on the use of data must be made clear to the subjects and subsequently strictly adhered to by the researcher'. Thus, the fulfilment of any pledge of confidentiality is an important dimension of accountability in research.

It is relatively easy to promise confidentiality of personal information which is collected in the course of a research project when subjects are part of a large sample and the data are quantitative in nature and, as such, reduced to collective numerical results. In such research – typically a survey – it is almost impossible for individual subjects to be identified in the final report. Nevertheless, this needs to be explained carefully to a potential subject who, unfamiliar with the process of data analysis, may not understand how personal information will be reduced to anonymity. Reassurance must also be given about how such data will be stored safely in the interim, for example under a code number rather than by name. Such reassurance is particularly important if very personal or controversial data are being collected, or if the research participants are (or feel) especially vulnerable. This may be the case, for example, when a study is concerned with people who have HIV infection or AIDS, or when patients are being invited by a researcher to be openly critical of the care they have received, or when nursing students still on course are being asked to evaluate their education programme.

The confidentiality of data gathered for research is much more difficult to guarantee in the case of a small sample or a setting-specific study. When the sample is small, personal data are less easy to reduce to anonymity, and in a time-specific research report an individual subject could conceivably be identified on the basis of even a limited number of straightforward details such as age, sex, occupation and medical diagnosis. Similarly, it can be difficult to conceal the identity of the location of a setting-specific study. It does not take too much detective work for a reader to track down a study location when, for example, it is described by an Edinburgh-based researcher as a 20-bedded male surgical ward in a large, local teaching hospital. Better, in my view, that pledges of confidentiality and anonymity are not given in such cases. It may well be that individual subjects and staff in particular settings will have no objection to being potentially identifiable in the research report. Whatever is decided, the researcher must be able to exercise accountability for the agreed procedures regarding the protection of confidential information which is collected for purposes of the research.

Being accountable when anonymity cannot be assured

Protecting the confidentiality of data collected in the course of a small-sample qualitative research study, however, is inherently difficult. It is possible that the researcher will be unable to guarantee anonymity, and this must be cleared in advance with the informants so that they consent to participation knowing that their accounts may be personally identifiable. In such cases, the researcher's accountability to the subjects is put to the most stringent of tests.

The personal dilemmas and discomfort that may be experienced by the researcher in such a situation are described by Bergum (1991) who undertook a phenomenological study of the real-life experiences of women in the transition through pregnancy, childbirth and early mothering. Her data derive from a series of conversations over time with six women. Bergum writes about the tension for a phenomenological researcher between the 'inner person' and the 'outer activities'. She reflects that 'the ethical commitments to these women permeated my mind and my actions throughout the study and still continue....Using their stories for my research purposes binds me to them in a way that goes beyond the technical considerations of how to handle the raw data of research'. Bergum also points out that in the published version of the study the women are not 'anonymous' to themselves and their words are 'available to (them) for continued reflection'. Thus, in a study such as this, private lives become public, and personal development is recorded for all time.

In qualitative studies it is sometimes the practice for the researcher to return the subjects' accounts to them for scrutiny. In doing so, the researcher is choosing to exercise accountability at a personal level to each of the participants in a way that does not occur in other forms of research. In principle, however, the same degree of personal accountability to subjects is present (theoretically, at least) in all research. The fact that research subjects generally do not have the opportunity to scrutinize and challenge the researcher's account and interpretation of the data does not lessen the researcher's responsibility to report the data truthfully, and thereby to fulfil their final responsibility in the process of accountability to the research participants.

Accountability to research 'gatekeepers'

Although potential participants in nursing and health services research are protected from exploitation by the requirement that a researcher obtains their personal consent to involvement, there is prior protection afforded by 'gatekeepers', through whom researchers must negotiate access before approaching potential subjects. This is necessary even when the proposed research has gained the approval of a funding body and of the relevant research ethics committee(s).

Who are the 'gatekeepers'?

'Gatekeepers' control a researcher's access to potential subjects or a site or information; in nursing research access to all three is usually required. In the health service, both practitioners and managers can act as gatekeepers. Indeed, access to these personnel may have to be sought in the first instance from higher authority. In Scotland, for example, it has been expected that the Chief Area Nursing Officer of the health board concerned should be the first line of approach when a nurse wishes to discuss a proposed research project with managers in the chosen site. In the case of research involving nursing students, the relevant college principal or head of department may act as a gatekeeper. Having obtained their permission, the researcher then pursues access downwards through the hierarchy.

This can be a time-consuming process, but it does provide protection for patients and staff. Quite reasonably, in their interests, a manager acting as a gatekeeper may rule that the entry of a researcher into a particular clinical area at a particular time and for a particular purpose is not acceptable. Thus, a request for research access may be refused. One assumes that such a managerial decision will have taken due account of the views of the ward sister and senior medical staff, and indeed that their views would carry most weight in the case of research to be conducted in their clinical area.

In some hospitals or areas, all requests for research access are now considered centrally by a research committee. In others, the researcher is expected to negotiate directly with managers and then with those who will be most immediately concerned with the research. Either way, there should be the expectation that all requests for access to conduct scientifically sound and justifiable research will be received sympathetically and assessed objectively. There is no justification for research access to be denied on the basis of a manager's whim or a ward sister's general lack of interest in research, or a doctor's refusal to accept that nursing research (or, indeed, any kind of research other than a randomized clinical trial) is a legitimate activity.

Some of the influences that affect the decision-making of gatekeepers are discussed by Mander (1992b) in the light of her own experiences in seeking access for a study of midwives' care of mothers whose babies were relinquished for adoption. Although she won the support of midwife managers with ease, some social workers were less cooperative. Like one of the research ethics committees involved, a hospital social worker failed to appreciate the relevance of the study to midwifery; and social workers in a local authority agency were not prepared to allow access to mothers contemplating relinquishment of their babies on grounds that the research would add further stress to an already very stressful situation. Mander advises that, when deciding whether or not to permit research access, the gatekeepers should recognize when their own experience is lacking or their views are based on mere assumptions. In such cases, she suggests, 'they should take advantage of the opportunity to draw on the expertise of those with different or more wide-ranging experience'.

Changing relationships with gatekeepers

In the current climate of encouragement for more collaboration between researchers and service-based personnel in the NHS, it is likely that the process of negotiation for research access will become less rather than more difficult. As managers and practitioners become more aware of the importance attached to research in the health service, they are likely to become more positive about facilitating it. It is likely, too, that the planning of research will more commonly become a joint enterprise. Thus, it will become less common for a researcher to finalize a research protocol and then begin the process of seeking access 'from cold'.

This should not mean, however, that health service managers and practitioners will become lax as gatekeepers. Although, wrongly, they may abuse their power, the gatekeepers will always have a very important role to play in safeguarding the interests of patients and the service by denying access for research which is time-wasting, scientifically unsound or ethically questionable. Hopefully, with the benefit of closer relationships with researchers, health service staff will be better informed about research and, as a result, better able to respond to requests for access on the basis of knowledge and experience rather than intuition or emotion.

Will the advent of the health-care 'market' change the relationship between gatekeepers and researchers? It might, at least in the short term, and not necessarily for the better. In the market scenario, Trusts are operating 'in competition' with each other and there is a split between the purchasers and the providers of health care. Certainly, it is in the interests of the providers, for the purposes of 'selling' their services to purchasers, to have research-based information that supports and explains their activities. Negative or equivocal research findings, however, might be seen as less than helpful, and provider units might be wary of supporting research which may produce results showing one Trust to be performing better than another, although the purchasers will of course be keenly interested in this.

It is conceivable that Trusts may become less willing to grant access for independent research which may produce findings that could disadvantage them in the health-care market. Trusts may therefore choose to rely increasingly on in-house research, or commissioned work over which internal control of results can be retained. Another possibility is that a Trust would continue to grant access to independent researchers but with conditions attached that limit the researcher's freedom to publish and, thereby, publicize the results.

It will be interesting to see how the role of research gatekeepers changes with the advent of the internal market in health care. If there is the kind of change envisaged, it will interesting too to see how central research grant-giving bodies will react if Trusts do become less willing to give access for publicly funded, multicentre studies, or at least less willing for the results of such research to be made public.

The researcher's accountability to gatekeepers

In the same way as a researcher has ongoing and specific accountability to their sponsor and the research ethics committee, there is continuing accountability to the research gatekeepers even after access has been granted. Access will have been granted on the basis of an agreed plan of action (i.e. the specified 'plan of investigation', as in the formal research protocol). The researcher is therefore bound to work within that agreed plan and, in exercising accountability, should not extend beyond the boundaries of that agreement and must adhere closely to the agreed procedures (for example the procedure for obtaining informed voluntary consent).

Very often, for reasons beyond the control of the researcher, the research plan has to be modified in the course of the project. For example, the sampling procedure that was piloted may not be working because the patient population of the study setting has changed as a consequence of a new admissions policy within the hospital. Or, perhaps, the method of non-participant observation which had been developed for use in the practice nurse's clinic in a health centre is proving to be too intrusive, even although it had been acceptable to staff and patients when piloted. In other cases, it might be that the promised cooperation of staff (for example to randomize a nursing intervention) is impossible to maintain because of new pressures or the introduction of new working methods within the ward. In such cases the researcher has the choice of abandoning the project or changing strategy. Either way, the decision must be made in consultation with the gatekeepers (and then with the approval of the sponsor) if the researcher's accountability to those in positions of authority is to be maintained.

And, of course, on completion of the work, the researcher should provide the gatekeepers with an account of the research findings. This may have to await the 'go-ahead' of the sponsor and it may require a modified form of reporting in order to preserve promised confidentiality to patients or staff, who may be recognized by insiders although they are impossible to identify from the outside. On this point, the RCN Ethical Guidelines for Nursing Research emphasize that 'any promises of anonymity or confidentiality given to the participants by the researcher must be respected also by the nurse commissioning or agreeing to a study being carried out'. 'No attempt should be made', the guidelines continue, 'to probe data or results in order to identify any individual, instance or place which has been concealed deliberately by the researcher'. Nurses in positions of authority where research is carried out are also advised that 'deviations from expected practice uncovered in the course of research should not be used by managers for punitive purposes although remedial actions would be expected to follow'. Thus by this analysis the researcher's accountability to the research participants takes priority.

Accountability to co-researchers

Most nursing research in the United Kingdom to date has been in the form of one-off, one-person studies. It is a sign of a developing maturity that more work is being done on a teamwork basis. In the academic nursing departments there has been a trend towards collective, collaborative research activity (Butterworth 1991). This is certainly the more common model in both science and social science disciplines, in which research is a well-established activity and where individual research projects are set within an ongoing, coordinated programme.

In the health service there is now an ever-increasing interest in multidisciplinary research. Nurses have a key role to play in this, not just as participants but also as initiators. Each member of the multidisciplinary research team is accountable to co-researchers.

The UKCC Code of Professional Conduct recognizes that teamwork adds a special dimension to the notion of personal accountability in nursing practice. The code (paragraph 5) expects that a nurse will 'work in a collaborative and cooperative manner with health-care professionals and others involved in providing care, and recognize their particular contributions within the care team'. The same principle can be taken to apply to accountability in the sphere of research.

The long-standing traditions and day-to-day tensions that make the ideals of multidisciplinary collaboration and cooperation so difficult to achieve in the context of healthcare practice are perhaps not as evident in the world of research. For a start, a research team is generally self-established, whereas members of a health-care team seldom have the opportunity to choose their colleagues. Furthermore, a research team has a much clearer and narrower remit and, in the form of stated research aims, a common goal which has been mutually agreed. Unlike a health-care team, a research team drives the work rather than being driven by external demand.

Nevertheless, there is the same demand for its members to recognize and respect each other's particular contributions. This is always taxing for individuals whose experiences and perspectives have been shaped by very different backgrounds. Not surprisingly, a doctor whose training and experience has been mainly in the realm of experimental research is bound to find it difficult to see the value of a 'soft' qualitative component in the research plan which the medical sociologist member of the team insists should be included. Neither of them may be as concerned as the nurse member about the practicalities of conducting the proposed project in a busy hospital ward, or about the demands of participation on sick, anxious patients. In turn, the nurse member of the team may be much more concerned with outcomes of care as perceived by the patients, and much less concerned than the health economist member with measuring the costs of that care. The process of planning a multidisciplinary research project requires time and, with it, a genuine willingness on the part of all members of the team to respect and accommodate each others' knowledge and experience.

Each member of the research team has different professional traditions and values to uphold. Nurses, in the words of the UKCC Code of Professional Conduct, are expected to 'uphold and enhance the good standing and reputation of the (nursing) professions'. By ensuring that the nursing dimensions of multi-disciplinary research are rigorously addressed, a nurse researcher is responding to that expectation and is exercising professional accountability.

Accountability to (and of) the profession

Like nurses in any sphere of professional practice, nurse researchers can be considered to be accountable to their peers: i.e. to the profession at large. It would have to be said that nurse researchers have not been held in particularly high esteem by the profession. They have been criticized for being 'ivory-towered' and out of touch with the real world of nursing. The topics of their research have been described as irrelevant and there has been much criticism of their perceived inability to communicate their findings in ways that are mean-ingful to practising nurses. For their part, researchers have retaliated by criticiz-ing the profession's lack of interest in research. The so-called gap between research and practice (and between researchers and practitioners) became a focus of concern in the 1980s.

The need for, and the difficulty of, improving relationships between the doers and the consumers of research is not unique to nursing. This is recognized as a challenge in all health professions and, indeed, in other areas, such as science and technology.

Changing relationships

In nursing, in recent years, there has been an evident improvement in the rela-tionship between the doers and the consumers of research. There is no doubt that nurse researchers have become very aware of the need for their research to have (and be seen to have) direct relevance to practice and service delivery issues, and for the findings to be reported in ways that nursing colleagues find interesting and meaningful to their everyday work.

For their part, practising nurses have become more appreciative of the contri-bution (and limitations) of research as, gradually, education at basic and post-basic levels has improved the extent of research awareness and knowledge throughout the profession. Research has now become a component of job descriptions in nursing and, as a result, practising nurses and nurses in management have come to appreciate that nurse researchers have expertise which is otherwise in short supply in the profession.

The development of this mutual appreciation is a welcome trend. Some successful initiatives in collaborative working have been reported (for example Tierney and Taylor 1991). It is just these sorts of interactive relationships that are encouraged in the new Research and Development Strategy for the NHS.

Towards shared accountability for research

As the gap between research and practice continues to close it can be expected that the profession will come to see itself as sharing accountability for nursing research with its researchers. In the past it may have been reasonable for nurse researchers to be blamed for the lack of impact of research, or its lack of relevance, but this is no longer an appropriate stance for the profession to adopt.

It was argued at the beginning of the chapter that any accountable profession must assume responsibility for the ongoing development of its knowledge base. It follows, therefore, that it is the profession's responsibility to ensure that its infrastructure supports research; that it possesses an adequate research capability; and that the research undertaken is relevant, and is disseminated and utilized effectively.

The formulation of the Strategy for Research in Nursing, Midwifery and Health Visiting (discussed earlier) is evidence that the profession has taken on this responsibility. Indeed, the task force that formulated the strategy saw itself as having some direct accountability for the uptake of its recommendations. It pledged to review progress with the implementation of the strategy a year or so after its publication, and further steps will presumably be taken if its recommendations are not being actively pursued.

Further, built into the strategy, the task force spelt out the respective responsibilities for research of managers, teachers, practitioners and researchers. Also, in 1993, nursing's professional organization in the United Kingdom, the RCN, established a Research Committee with the purpose of strengthening and coordinating the RCN's contribution to, and support of, research in nursing.

These are important landmarks in the profession's development in terms of its commitment to research. Thus, in the 1990s, accountability for research is being seen, for the first time, as a collective responsibility of the profession as a whole and not just its researchers.

Accountability to the wider public

Since an awareness of the importance of research in nursing is relatively new, it is not surprising that it does not feature largely in the public image of nursing. Most lay people still perceive nursing as being an essentially practical occupation, more in need of kind hearts than clever heads. This view seems to be common even among people in similarly practical fields of work, such as engineering, computing, accountancy and dentistry, in which the role of research is taken for granted.

It is no wonder, really, that lay people have such a poor appreciation of the nature and relevance of nursing research. Rarely has there been any mass media coverage in this country of the results of a nursing research study. I remember being pleased but startled when I read a magazine report of a piece of research I had done concerning the experiences and information needs of women who were undergoing chemotherapy for breast cancer (Tierney *et al.* 1993). Why should I have been startled? In almost every daily newspaper there are reports of medical and scientific research. Every year, there is detailed news coverage of the proceedings of the British Psychological Society's scientific meeting. Why has nursing research not been similarly reported in the public domain? This is something that should be remedied if we want to improve public recognition of the role of research in nursing and, indeed, of the whole changing nature of nursing practice and nursing education. The nursing profession has long enjoyed the support of the British public and, in the current era of health service reform, the continuation of that support is vital. The place and importance of research in nursing needs to be explained. Many members of the public may be unaware that nursing services are the largest single item of health service expenditure. If there was a greater awareness of this fact, it is likely that the public would appreciate the crucial role that research can (and needs to) play in demonstrating the worth and value of nursing. Indeed, the public may be quicker than the profession itself has been to appreciate that such research is, *a priori*, a responsibility of a publicly accountable profession.

TENSIONS OF MULTIPLE ACCOUNTABILITY

Accountability in research has been examined in relation to a number of different parties: the sponsor, research ethics committees, research participants, gatekeepers, co-researchers, the profession and the wider public. Some of these parties are in positions of authority (for example the sponsor and the gatekeepers), whereas others are in positions of equality (for example co-researchers) or dependence (i.e. participating patients). Depending on their positions, the researcher's accountability derives from duty or dueness and, correspondingly, it is more or less regulated by formal mechanisms or ethical conventions. When an individual is required to exercise different types of accountability to a number of parties – as, in terms of this analysis, is the case for a nurse researcher – there are, inevitably, inherent tensions.

The tensions of multiple accountability in nursing research are probably felt most acutely by nurses who are engaged in on-the-job research. In such a situation the key tensions arise from the individual's dual role as nurse *and* researcher. In relation to clinical responsibilities, the nurse is accountable to the employing organization through the usual channels. In relation to parallel research responsibilities, there may be formal accountability to an external sponsor or supervisor. Conflicts of interest may arise.

The RCN Ethical Guidelines for Nursing Research offer useful advice for nurses in such a position. They state:

'When research is undertaken in the context of an organizational structure, it is important to clarify in advance the responsibilities of the researcher within the organization, the lines of communication and the means of settling any conflicts of interest which may arise.'

Conflicts of interest do arise. How does the nurse fulfil accountability to meet the completion deadline set by the research sponsor when the pressing demands of clinical work eat into the time that has been agreed for the research? Can the nurse always fulfil accountability to the research subjects in terms of confidentiality of data when that same data may be recognized as being potentially crucial to the patient's medical or nursing care? What does the nurse do when research uncovers colleagues acting unethically or negligently? And when a patient, as research subject, breaks down in distress is it possible to maintain the detached stance expected of a researcher, or should the nurse offer the type of professional counsel which would be appropriate to the role of practitioner?

The role of a nurse researcher who is not also carrying clinical responsibilities is, in contrast, less complicated. On this, the RCN guidelines state that 'the nurse who is undertaking a research project in an exclusively research role has no responsibility for the service, care, treatment or advice given to patients or clients unless stipulated within the design of the research'. In theory this is perfectly correct, and a nurse researcher would not be held accountable for patient care. The guidelines make clear that 'any intervention in a professional capacity should be confined to situations in which a patient or client requires to be protected or rescued from danger'.

In practice, however, it can be difficult to decide what constitutes 'danger'. Reasonably, a nurse researcher may feel that it is better to err on the safe side and to act as a nurse rather than be criticized later for foolishly maintaining a 'stand-off' position as a researcher. After all, the first rule in the UKCC Code of Professional Conduct states that a nurse must 'act always in such a manner as to promote and safeguard the interests and wellbeing of patients and clients'. Is a researcher who is also a nurse ever expected to act at odds with this?

In a hospital ward, or other environment in which the research subjects are patients under care, it is usually easy for the nurse researcher, without breaching confidentiality, to find a way of conveying anxieties to staff or encouraging patients themselves to pass on information that the researcher feels, in the patient's interest, should be known to staff. In one study for which I had supervisory responsibility, the research assistant who was interviewing elderly patients in a hospital ward kept coming across patients who, when asked, reported that they were suffering from pain, sometimes to a considerable degree. Sticking closely to her instructions to behave as a researcher, she had not conveyed her concern to the staff. It was not in the interests of the research to alert staff to the apparent need for better pain management because the aim of the study was to obtain baseline data prior to the introduction of potential improvements. As nurses, however, we did not feel we could continue to collect evidence of inadequate pain control without alerting the ward staff, and so this was done.

Much more difficult dilemmas arose in the course of a study which involved interviews at home with elderly patients who had been recently discharged from hospital (Tierney *et al.* 1992). An experienced health visitor was employed to undertake these interviews and it was emphasized that her role was as a researcher. Contingency plans were agreed in case, in her professional judgement, she considered any of the subjects to be in difficulty and in need of care or attention. The main strategy was that she would advise the elderly person (or the carer) to contact the GP. If they were unwilling to do so, she would ask their permission to contact the GP herself. There were a number of the elderly people who were found to be in dire straits, and the contingency plans proved to be satisfactory in most cases. There were instances, however, when the researcher did not consider there was real danger but, as a health visitor, she felt compelled to offer professional advice and, occasionally, to give hands-on care. There were also circumstances which we had not anticipated. For example, there were occasions when there was no answer when the researcher arrived at the prearranged time to undertake the interview. Did she just go away and bemoan the loss of an interview and the waste of time? No; as a health visitor with a keenly developed sense of professional accountability she did whatever was necessary to ensure that the elderly person was safely elsewhere or, if in the house, was not in danger or in need of help.

These examples are not especially dramatic. They do illustrate, however, that there are tensions for the nurse researcher – irrespective of which is the primary role – between accountability as a researcher and accountability as a nurse.

CONCLUSION

Accountability is a notion which is simple to define but difficult to elucidate in terms of its operationalization in everyday practice. Before setting out to write this chapter I had not had occasion to think in a structured or reflective way about the scope and meaning of accountability in the context of nursing research, and it was interesting and instructive to have to do so. Although I had always been aware of the significance and pervasiveness of the notion of accountability in relation to research, its centrality to everyday research practice had not struck me before. I also had not appreciated, consciously at least, that accountability in research is so inextricably bound up with ethics, intra- and interprofessional issues and, wider still, with nursing's public accountability. In these respects, accountability in nursing research is no different from account-ability in any other sphere of nursing. Without doubt, many of the issues and themes in this chapter will have been raised already, albeit in various guises, in earlier parts of this book.

14

Accountability in nursing education

Diane Marks-Maran

INTRODUCTION

Any profession needs to define and clarify its goals, set its standards and monitor its performance. In doing so it accounts for its practice to all those who have
an interest or stake in that profession. Accountability in nursing has been examined extensively in the literature and has been high on the agenda of the statutory bodies and professional trade unions for nurses, midwives and health
visitors.

Accountability in nursing education, however, has not received the same
level of attention and interest. This chapter will address the following issues:
changes to accountability in nursing education; new accountability issues and
new 'stakeholders'; resolving the accountability conflicts in nursing education;
and issues related to teaching accountability.

CHANGING ACCOUNTABILITY AND NURSING EDUCATION

Historically, the interested parties in accountability in nursing and midwifery
education have been described quite simply. Roch (1988), for instance, identified that midwifery education was accountable to students, consumers of health
care (patients/clients), managers of the service and statutory bodies.

More recently, the English National Board (ENB 1993) has redefined to
whom the key interested parties in nursing education are accountable: the
national boards and the UKCC; individual institutions of higher education
where education is linked; purchasers of education, students, academic and clinical staff, who contribute to its development; and patient/client groups, who are

the ultimate recipients of education. It could be argued, however, that not all of the above have the mechanisms, power or opportunity to call nursing education to account or to exact accountability from it.

In the 1990s two significant changes to nursing and midwifery education are also influencing, and indeed changing, the face of educational accountability. These are the move of nursing and midwifery education into higher education, and the purchaser–provider split arising from the creation of an education market. These two aspects are changing what nursing is accountable for and to whom it is accountable.

The integration of nursing into higher education

Increased accountability by institutions of higher education is of increasing public concern. New mechanisms have been introduced that require universities to demonstrate both financial and educational accountability (Williams and Loder 1990; Perry 1990; Powell 1991). As nursing and midwifery education integrates into higher education, both the 'who?' and the 'what?' of accountability alter to require that account is rendered to new interested parties in higher education, funding bodies and regulatory bodies. Nursing and midwifery education is now accountable to university validation and review boards and mechanisms with regard to the quality of academic course provision. This is in addition to its accountability to professional statutory bodies.

The purchaser–provider split in education

As a result of the relevant NHS reform working papers for education in the United Kingdom, there will now be a separation of those who provide nursing and midwifery education and those who purchase it. The new arrangements can be summarized as follows:

- Colleges of nursing and midwifery are amalgamating to form larger institutions which will integrate completely into a university. The nature and extent of this integration varies between health regions.
- Health regions will act as funding agencies for education provision.
- Different health regions have made different arrangements for how education will be purchased. For example, some regions have been geographically divided into consortia, with each consortium made up of the health-care provider units within that geographical area. Regions or consortia then decide which universities, colleges of nursing or midwifery will be awarded educational contracts for pre- and post-registration nursing and midwifery.
- Regions or consortia can award all educational contracts to one institution. Conversely, they can divide the contracts and award different contracts to different institutions.
- Only certain courses will be contracted in this way. These include statutory

preregistration nursing courses (e.g. Project 2000, 3-year preregistration, 18-month post-registration midwifery courses) and post-basic, specialist clinical courses (e.g. the traditional 6-month English National Board (ENB) clinical courses).

● Courses other than these that colleges offer will be 'sold' to individual units, individual health-care professionals who wish to undertake them, or to any other purchasers on the open market.

These two new dimensions, integration into higher education and the purchaser–provider split, are bringing about changes in the nature of account-ability in nursing education. The 'who?' of accountability has altered to include new bodies who are interested in different aspects of the educational quality for which they call nursing education to account.

In summary, course development and provision now need to suit purchaser requirements, and purchasers will be free to contract for education provision elsewhere if the education provider cannot appropriately account for the quality of education provision. In addition, nursing and midwifery education is now accountable to new bodies for academic quality and research. These changes represent an addition to both the 'who?' and the 'what?' of accountability. How nursing and midwifery education renders account in this new scenario will be discussed below.

NEW ISSUES OF ACCOUNTABILITY FOR NURSING AND MIDWIFERY EDUCATION

Demonstrating accountability

The new accountability issues that have emerged as a result of the changes in nursing and midwifery education have an impact on how colleges of nursing and midwifery go about their business. The way in which colleges demonstrate accountability is also having to change. The major issues which will be discussed here are course planning and delivery, academic validation, monitor-ing and annual review processes, setting education standards, and monitoring the achievement of standards meeting conflicting stakeholder demands for accountability.

Course planning and delivery

Prior to integration and linking with higher education, course planning and course documentation involved meeting the requirements of the relevant National Board. These were largely professional and educational requirements, as course approval did not particularly rely on judging the academic level of the programme. Integration into higher education has brought new issues to those who plan and deliver nursing and midwifery programmes. Course planners, for instance, have had to learn how to meet the academic requirements of higher education, as courses and programmes are jointly validated in relation to both professional as well as academic standards.

Colleges of nursing and midwifery now need to justify their courses at appropriate academic levels in terms of outcomes, assessment, content and teaching methods. Superimposed on this is the need for course planners to meet the requirements of purchasers, who are calling colleges of nursing and midwifery to account for other aspects of their work. Purchasers are now beginning to articulate exactly what they require from colleges: they wish to know what those who complete courses can demonstrate in terms of what they know and can do.

Achievement-led outcome-based learning

An achievement-led college is a holistic concept based on the assumption that everything a college does has a bearing upon individual achievement (Shackleton 1990) and that the institution – its structures, its resources, its philosophy and its educational provision – should have as its central tenet and starting point one concept: individual development and achievement. Shackleton (1990) suggested that many colleges focus on the syllabus and the needs or wants of the teachers, and that the students are often secondary and are expected to adjust themselves to the curriculum. In short, in most institutions the focus is on teaching rather than learning.

Outcome-based programmes are a natural adjunct to an achievement-led approach. An outcome-based programme is one where specific targets, in the form of learning outcomes, are clearly identified at each stage. In nursing and midwifery education, the learning outcomes are largely service identified and represent, in measurable terms, what knowledge and skills the nursing or midwifery service requires of the person who has completed that programme.

Once learning outcomes are identified throughout a programme, decisions are made between education and service as to how the agreed learning outcomes will be assessed. This may be through theoretical assessment, clinical assessment or both. The remaining aspects of the programme – content and teaching/learning methods – are then carefully selected in order to enable students to achieve those outcomes.

Students may select the learning methods most appropriate for their own achievement needs. The college is accountable to the student for providing the resources that will enable them to achieve their targets (outcomes) and to the nursing service for producing nurses who can function in a way that meets service requirements, as identified in the learning outcomes.

There is a movement within the higher education sector generally to develop courses which are learning outcome-led (Otter 1990). Such an approach will enable colleges of nursing and midwifery to satisfy competing demands for accountability from universities and from purchasers of education in the health service. Outcome-based course planning can be described as educational planning which is service directed but educationally led. It enables the vocational needs of the service to sit alongside academic requirements through learning outcomes which can be written specifically for differing academic levels.

Levels of learning outcomes

Learning outcomes can be divided into various levels. A level 1 outcome, for example, might only expect a student to be assessed at a certain cognitive level, e.g. to be able to describe or compare and contrast, or to apply foundation principles of knowledge to practice. An example of a level 1 learning outcome might be: 'Understand and apply the principles and practice of health promotion in the practitioner's work setting' (ENB 1991). A level 2 learning outcome, on the other hand, would expect the student to be able to do more than simply describe or apply foundation knowledge to practice. Instead, a level 2 learning might be written as follows: 'Provide care which applies specialist knowledge and skills to meet the needs of a client population' (ENB 1991). In this outcome the expectation is that students will be able to demonstrate that they have in-depth knowledge and can apply this knowledge to practice.

A level 3 outcome might expect students to demonstrate higher cognitive skills and abilities, e.g. synthesis, critical analysis and evaluation, or to apply specialist knowledge and skills over a wider client group, such as an entire caseload, or as a team leader. An example of a level 3 learning outcome might be: 'Critically examine and promote change in delivery of care in the light of research findings specific to the client group' (ENB 1991).

In summary, an achievement-led outcome-based approach allows for professional, purchaser and academic requirements to be drawn together, thus decreasing competing and conflicting accountability for the education provider. Assessment schemes and methods can be designed which test the achievement of learning outcomes at all levels. This is often achieved through work-related projects which address a real clinical need or problem in projects which are jointly agreed by student, teacher and clinical manager, and which fulfil an academic requirement. The National Health Service Training Department (NHSTD) health pick-up packages are examples of this approach which, among other things, decrease the competing accountability requirements of various interested parties.

Validation, monitoring and review

Another duality faced by colleges of nursing and midwifery is the competing requirements of joint professional validation. The criteria against which statutory bodies call nursing education to account are different from those applied by a university, in terms of the nature of the information required regarding course content and validation, and also in terms of aspects such as assessment.

Traditionally, some universities which have run nursing programmes have had both theoretical and clinical assessments. In many the inclusion of a clinical assessment was required in order to fulfil the expectations of the statutory bodies and the profession. However, it was often the case that the degree classification was only determined by the theoretical work of the student. With the shift towards competing demands of accountability the purchasers of education are likely to want clinical skills to have at least equal value to theoretical knowledge. Some university-based nursing colleges are now creating programmes which are validated so that this is indeed the case (Queen Charlotte's College 1992).

Professional statutory bodies have different interests and agendas from universities when it comes to validation and course monitoring and review. For example, some universities use nationally agreed performance indicators as the criteria for accounting for academic performance and quality (CNAA 1992). The English National Board, on the other hand, has different criteria to determine the performance of colleges (ENB 1993). One way of marrying these two aspects of accountability is through educational standard setting.

Educational standard setting

As colleges of nursing and midwifery integrate into higher education and, at the same time, enter the purchaser–provider marketplace, ways of accounting for the quality of education provision will need to be created that satisfy both.

All interested parties have their own ideas of what they believe counts as quality, and will call colleges to account for these. One way in which colleges can merge competing requirements, and thereby render account to both sets of expectations, is to work with both sets of 'stakeholders' in setting and agreeing educational standards.

Jointly written and agreed educational standards which are turned into measurable criteria become the benchmark against which the college can account to all interested parties for the quality of its education provision. Educational standards can then form the basis for monitoring and review of the college and its courses.

This section has concentrated on some of the key accountability issues facing nursing education in the 1990s. The major issues of dual accountability cover course planning and delivery, validation, monitoring and review. Two suggestions have been put forward as a way of bringing together the problem of competing accountability: the use of achievement-led outcomes-based approaches to course planning, and educational standard setting. The next section will focus on the concept of 'biculturalism' with regard to accountability in nursing education.

RESOLVING THE ACCOUNTABILITY CONFLICT: TOWARDS BICULTURALISM

Higher education has its own culture, its own norms, values and expectations. So too has the health service. Nursing education needs to be able to live comfortably with a foot in each culture. Kramer (1974), in examining the cultures of the 'ideal' versus the 'real' in nursing, coined the term 'biculturalism'. In the same way as the real world of nursing and the ideal world of nursing have conflicting values and practices, the expectations of higher education often conflict with the expectations of the health service regarding education. The conflict is not only about competing or differing values, norms and practices. It is also about competing notions of accountability and that for which nursing education is to be called to account.

Biculturalism, as regards accountability in nursing education, is the ability to get along within competing expectations without being totally absorbed by one or the other. It is the ability to render account adequately to competing sets of quality expectations, understanding the norms and values of each cultural system sufficiently with the ability to establish one's identity within each.

Biculturalism is the positive response to the conflicting accountabilities in nursing education today. There are also a number of potentially destructive alternatives to biculturalism, and these have been identified by Kramer (1974) as:

- rejecting one system of expectations and only accounting adequately to the demands of one culture. This may lead to purchasers perhaps being pleased with course provision but validating bodies withholding validation and approval due to problems of academic level. Conversely, it can lead to programmes that succeed at validation but are not attractive to purchasers;
- teachers leaving one culture completely to immerse themselves entirely in the other; this may take the form of teachers going back into clinical practice or entering the 'ivory tower' of academic study and research;
- rejecting both cultures and not getting involved in either, e.g. 'just putting in the hours';
- burning out;
- changing jobs frequently when accountability conflicts arise;
- leaving nursing and education completely for another career.

It is suggested that the move to achievement-led outcome-based approaches and joint educational standard setting and monitoring between all interested parties can be practical tools for becoming bicultural.

TEACHING AND LEARNING ACCOUNTABILITY

Apart from the theory and knowledge base surrounding accountability, which can be learned in any number of ways, it is suggested here that being able to practise and develop the ability to account for and justify one's own practice as a normal aspect of personal behaviour is most effectively learned through role modelling or mentorship, and through reflecting on practice.

Role modelling

Nurses learn many of their skills and professional behaviours from seeing how other, sometimes more senior, colleagues work. This is true for psychomotor skills and activities as well as for interpersonal behaviours. Teachers can act as role models for professional accountability in a number of ways.

First, as part of their own clinical practice teachers can demonstrate that they account to their patients, their students and their nursing and medical colleagues for their own nursing decisions. They can, when appropriate, also call others to account or to justify care decisions, especially when working with students in clinical practice. Learning accountability is about learning that to account for one's professional decisions is a normal part of professional behaviour, and involves examining and explaining why certain decisions were taken and why one option was chosen over all others. Therefore, the teacher acts as a role model for accountability, by first justifying their own decisions as a normal part of practice, and secondly by calling others to account as a normal part of their supervisory role.

Reflecting on practice

A second way in which accountability can be learned is through structured reflective activities between a supervisor and a less experienced nurse. Johns (1993) offers a model for structured reflection which can be used to facilitate students' reflection on incidents occurring in practice and to learn from them. The model involves describing an incident in detail using key questions, reflecting in a structured way on the incident and the action taken, identifying options and alternative actions which could have been taken and, finally, identifying the learning that has resulted from reflection. Using Johns' (1993) model, critical incidents specifically related to accountability can be examined and reflected upon and used as a learning tool.

The learning that results from reflecting on incidents involving accounting for nursing judgements should then enable the student to manage future incidents of accountability in a more confident and professional way. The role of the supervisor is to help the student through the process of reflection so that learning can take place.

CONCLUSION

This chapter has attempted to examine the issues of accountability in nursing education and how these are changing as a result of changes in the health service and the integration of nursing and midwifery education into higher education. Both these changes have led to a redefinition of accountability in nursing education, the identification of new interested parties with new demands and agendas, and an emergence of new accountability issues, such as those related to course planning, delivery and evaluation, validation monitoring and review. Finally, two suggestions are put forward: that the dual accountabilities to health service demands and higher education demands will lead to a state of conflict for teachers; and that Kramer's notion of biculturalism is a way of responding to this conflict positively; outcome-based programmes are suggested as a practical way of moving forwards with feet in both camps.

By bringing key interested parties together in terms of planning outcome-based programmes and through joint educational standard setting and monitoring, the conflicts arising from dual and multiple accountabilities can be minimized.

References

Abel-Smith B (1960) *A History of the Nursing Profession,* Heinemann, London

Adler M and Asquith S (1981) Discretion and power, in *Discretion and Welfare*, eds M Adler and S Asquith, Heinemann, London, 9–32

Aggleton PJ and Chalmers HA (1986) *Nursing Models and the Nursing Process,* Macmillan, London

Alderman C (1993) A family loss. *Nursing Standard,* **7**(27), 18–19

Alderson P (1990) *Choosing for Children,* Oxford University Press, Oxford

Alderson P (1993) *Childrens' Consent to Surgery,* Open University Press, Milton Keynes

Alexander C, Weisman C and Chase G (1981) Evaluating primary nursing in hospitals: examination of effects on nursing staff. *Medical Care,* **19**, 80–89

Allmark P and Klarzynski R (1992) The case against nurse advocacy. *British Journal of Nursing,* **2**, 33–36

Althusser L (1971) *Lenin and Philosophy and Other Essays,* New Left Books, London

Altschul A (1972) *Patient–Nurse Interaction,* Churchill Livingstone, Edinburgh

Angell (1990) Prisoners of technology: the case of Nancy Cruzan. *New England Journal of Medicine,* **332**(17), 1226–1228

Anonymous (1992) Skill mix report slammed. *Health Visitor,* **66**, 39

Archard D (1993) *Children: Rights and Childhood,* Routledge, London

Aristotle (1962) *Nicomachean Ethics,* Bobbs-Merrill Educational Publishing Ltd, Indianapolis

Armitage S (1990) Research utilisation in practice. *Nurse Education Today,* **10**, 10–15

ASC (Action for Sick Children) (1987) *Caring for Children in the Health Services,* Action for Sick Children, London

Atkinson P (1977) The reproduction of medical knowledge, in *Health Care and Health Knowledge*, ed R Dingwall, Croom Helm, London, 85–86

Audit Commission (1992) *Community Care: Managing the Cascade of Care,* HMSO, London

Bailey R and Clarke M (1989) *Stress and Coping in Nursing,* Chapman and Hall, London

Baly M (1986) *Florence Nightingale and the Nursing Legacy,* Croom Helm, London

Barker P (1982) *Behaviour Therapy Nursing,* Croom Helm, London

Barker W (1993) Patch and practice: specialist roles for health visitors. *Health Visitor,* **66**, 200–203

Barker W and Anderson R (1988) *The Child Development Programme: an Evaluation of Process and Outcomes,* Early Childhood Development Unit, University of Bristol

Baruch G (1981) Moral tales: parents' stories of encounters with the health professions. *Sociology of Health and Illness,* **3**, 275–295

Beck A (1976) *Cognitive Therapy and the Emotional Disorders*, Penguin, London

Beech B (1992) Rights and wrongs in maternity care. *Modern Midwife*, **2**, 8–10

Beecham L (1992) Role of health visitors in public health: report of Committee for Public Health Medicine and Community Health (BMA). *British Medical Journal*, **305**, 959

Bennett WL and Feldman MS (1981) *Reconstructing Reality in the Courtroom*, Tavistock, London

Benson ER (1990) Nineteenth century women, the neophyte nursing profession and the World's Columbian Exposition of 1893, in *Florence Nightingale and Her Era*, eds V Bullough, B Bullough and M P Stanton, Garland, New York, 108–122

Berger P and Luckmann T (1967) *The Social Construction of Reality*, Pelican, Harmondsworth

Bergman R (1981) Accountability: definitions and dimensions. *International Nursing Review*, **28**, 53–59

Bergum V (1991) Being a phenomenological researcher, in *Qualitative Nursing Research*, ed J M Morse, Sage Publications, London, 55–71

Billingham K (1991) Public health and the community. *Health Visitor*, **64**, 40–43

Binnie A, Bond S, Law G *et al.* (1984) *A Systematic Approach to Nursing Care*, Open University Press, Milton Keynes

Binnie A (1990) Proceedings of the Nursing Times Primary Nursing Conference, Hospitality Inn, Glasgow 18–19 July 1990

BJN (1903) *British Journal of Nursing,* 21 November, 409

BJN (1915a) *British Journal of Nursing*, 30 January (supplement), i

BJN (1915b) *British Journal of Nursing*, 27 March, 245

Black F (1992) *Primary Nursing: an Introductory Guide*, King's Fund Centre, London

Black N (1992) Research, audit, and education leading for health: responses. *British Medical Journal*, **304**, 698–700

Blackburn C (1992) *Poverty Profiling*, Health Visitors' Association, London

Blair F, Sparger G, Watts L and Thompson J (1982) Primary nursing in the emergency department: nurse–patient satisfaction. *Journal of Emergency Nursing*, **8**, 181–186

Bloor M and Fonkert JD (1982) Reality construction, reality exploration and treatment in two therapeutic communities. *Sociology of Health and Illness*, **4**, 125–140

Bluglass R (1983) *A Guide to the Mental Health Act 1983*, Churchill Livingstone, Edinburgh

Borst-Eilers E (1993) *To Treat or Not to Treat? Dilemmas Posed by the Hopelessly Ill.* Paper presented at the Royal Society of Edinburgh International Conference, Edinburgh 23–24 February 1993

Bond S, Bond J, Fowler P and Fall M (1991) Evaluating primary nursing. *Nursing Standard*, **5**(36) 35–39 (part 1); (37) 37–39 (part 2); (38) 36–39 (part 3)

Bowers L (1989) The significance of primary nursing. *Journal of Advanced Nursing*, **14**, 13–19

Brahams D (1981) Acquittal of paediatrician charged after death of infant with Down syndrome. *Lancet*, **2**, 1101–1102

Brewin TB (1986) Voluntary euthanasia. *Lancet*, **1**, 1085

British Medical Association (1988) *Euthanasia: Report of the BMA Working Party*, BMA, London

British Medical Association Medical Ethics Committee (1992) *Discussion Paper on Treatment of Patients in Persistent Vegetative State*, BMA, London

British Medical Association and Royal College of Nursing (1993) *Cardiopulmonary Resuscitation: a Statement from the BMA and RCN*, BMA and RCN, London

Brody H (1992) Assisted death – a compassionate response to a medical failure. *New England Journal of Medicine*, **327**(19), 1384–1389

Brooker C (1990) The application of the concept of expressed emotion to the role of the community psychiatric nurse: a research study. *International Journal of Nursing Studies*, **27**, 277–285

Brown JM, Kitson AL and McKnight TJ (1992) *Challenges in Caring: Explorations in Nursing and Ethics*, Chapman & Hall, London

Butterworth T (1991) Continuity in research and teaching. *Nursing Standard*, **5**(935), 31–36

Campbell AGM (1992) Baby Doe and forgoing life-sustaining treatment. Compassion, discrimination or medical neglect? in *Compelled Compassion: Government Intervention in the Treatment of Critically Ill Newborns*, eds A L Caplan, R H Blank and J C Merrick, Humana Press, New Jersey, 207–236

Carr-Saunders AM and Wilson PA (1933) *The Professions*, Clarendon Press, Oxford

Carter GB (1939) *A New Deal for Nurses*, Gollancz, London

Casey A (1993) Development and use of the partnership model of nursing care, in *Advances in Child Health Nursing*, eds A Glasper and A Tucker, Scutari, Harrow, 183–189

Central Health Services Council (1991) *Welfare of Children and Young People in Hospital*, HMSO, London

Chalmers K (1993) Searching for health needs: the work of health visiting. *Journal of Advanced Nursing*, **18**, 900–911

Champion R (1991) Educational accountability – what ho the 1990s! *Nurse Education Today*, **11**, 407–414

Chapman G (1987) *Text, Talk and Discourse: Nurses' Use of Language in a Therapeutic Community*. PhD thesis, University of London

Clifford C (1985) Helplessness: a concept applied to practice. *Intensive Care Nursing*, **1**, 19–24

Cook ET (1913) *The Life of Florence Nightingale, Vol 2*, Macmillan, London

Cook P (1990) Who's accountable? *Journal of District Nursing*, June, 18–20

Cooper J and Harpin V (1991) *This is Our Child,* Oxford University Press, Oxford

Copp G (1988) Professional accountability: the conflict. *Nursing Times*, **84**(43), 42–44

Cormack D (1976) *Psychiatric Nursing Observed*, Royal College of Nursing, London

Council for National Academic Awards (CNAA) (1992) *Academic Quality in Higher Education: a Guide to Good Practice*, CNAA, London

Cowley S (1993) Skill mix: value for whom? *Health Visitor*, **66**, 166–168

Cranford RE (1988) The persistent vegetative state: the medical reality (getting the facts straight). *Hasting Centre Report*, **18**(1), 27–32

Croog SH and Levine S (1977) *The Heart Patient Recovers*, Human Science Press, New York

Crossley T (1993) Too scared to care. Nursing Standard, **7**(40), 48–49

Cunningham G and Hiscock M (1992) *A Multidisciplinary Approach to Pain Management*, Royal Brompton National Heart and Lung Hospital, London

Curtin L (1982) Autonomy, accountability and nursing practice. *Topics in Clinical Nursing*, April, 7–13

Davidson B, Laan RV, Davis A *et al*. (1990) Ethical reasoning associated with the feeding of terminally ill elderly cancer patients. *Cancer Nursing*, **13**(5), 286–292

Davis AJ (1991) The sources of a practice code of ethics for nurses. *Journal of Advanced Nursing*, **16**, 1358–1362

Denzin NK (1989) *Interpretive Interactionism*, Sage, London

Department of Health (1990a) *Caring for People: Community Care in the Next Decade and Beyond*, HMSO, London

Department of Health (1990b) *Community Care Act*, HMSO, London

Department of Health (1990c) *General practice in the National Health Service: a new contract*, HMSO, London

Department of Health (1991a) *The Patient's Charter*, HMSO, London

Department of Health (1991b) *Research for Health: A Research and Development Strategy for the NHS*, Department of Health R and D Division, London

Department of Health (1992a) *Patient's Charter Citizen's Charter*, HMSO, London

Department of Health (1992b) *The Health of the Nation*, HMSO, London

Department of Health (1993a) *The Challenges for Nursing and Midwifery in the 21st Century*, HMSO, London

Department of Health (1993b) *Report of the Task Force on the Strategy for Research in Nursing, Midwifery and Health Visiting*, Department of Health R and D Division, London

Department of Health and Social Security (1986) *Neighbourhood Nursing: a Focus for Care* (Cumberlege report), HMSO, London

Dickinson E (1957) *Poems by Emily Dickinson*, Little, Brown and Co, Boston

Dingwall R, Rafferty A M and Webster C (1988) *An Introduction to the Social History of Nursing*, Routledge, London

Dock LL (1899) Nursing in England. *Nursing Record and Hospital World*, 11 November, 395–397

Dock LL (1901) *American Journal of Nursing*, 865

Dock LL (1912) *A History of Nursing, Vol 3*, Putnam, New York

Downe S (1989) Midwives alert! The times they are a-changin... *MIDIRS*, 12

Duff RS and Campbell AGM (1973) Moral and ethical dilemmas in the special care nursery. *New England Journal of Medicine*, **289**, 890–894

Dyer C (1985) The Gillick judgement, contraception and the under 16s: House of Lords Ruling. *British Medical Journal*, **291**, 1208–1209

Dyer C (1992) GMC tempers justice with mercy in Cox Case. *British Medical Journal*, **305**, 1311

Engel GV (1970) Professional autonomy and bureaucratic organisation. *Administrative Science Quarterly*, **15**, 12–215

English National Board (1991) *Framework for Continuing Professional Education for Nurses, Midwives and Health Visitors: a Guide to Implementation*, ENB, London

English National Board (1993) *Guidelines for Educational Audit*, ENB, London

Ersser S and Tutton E (1991) *Primary Nursing in Perspective*, Scutari Press, London

Etzioni A (1975) Epilogue: alternative conceptions of accountability, in *Accountability in Health Facilities*, ed H I Greenfield, Praeger, New York, 121–142

Evans A (1993) Accountability: a core concept for primary nursing. *Journal of Advanced Nursing*, **2**, 231–234

Expert Maternity Group (1993) *Changing childbirth*, HMSO, London

Fenwick Mrs Bedford (1887) Address to hospital matrons 10 December (reprinted). *British Journal of Nursing*, 15 May 1920, 288

Fenwick Mrs Bedford (1897) The better organisation of the nursing profession. *Nursing Record and Hospital World*, 6 November, 369–371 and 13 November, 389–391

Fenwick Mrs Bedford (1901A) The organisation and registration of nurses. Transactions of the Third International Congress of Nurses Pan-American Exposition, Buffalo 18–21 September, 339–340

Fenwick Mrs Bedford (1901B) A plea for the higher education of trained nurses. Transactions of the Third International Congress of Nurses Pan-American Exposition, Buffalo 18–21 September, 363–369

Flint C (1985) Trouble and strife. *Nursing Times*, **81**(45), 22

Flint C (1989) Requiem for midwifery. *MIDIRS*, 12

Flint C (1990) The demise of the midwifery profession. *Midwife Health Visitor and Community Nurse*, **26**, 66

Flint C and Poulengeris P (1987) *The Know Your Midwife Report*, South West Thames Regional Health Authority and Wellington Foundation, London

Foucault M (1979) *Discipline and Punish*, Peregrine, Harmondsworth

Foucault M (1982) The subject and power: afterword, in *Michel Foucault: Beyond Structuralism and Hermeneutics*, eds H L Dreyfus and P Rabinow, Harvester, Brighton, 2098–226

Fradd E (1990) Sharing accountability. *Paediatric Nursing*, **2**(3), 6–8

Freed EX (1975) Accountability in mental health care. *Journal of Nursing Administration*, **5**, 36–37

French P (1993) *Responsibility Matters*, Kansas University Press, Lawrence

Friedson E (1974) *The Professions and their Prospects*, Sage Publications, Beverly Hills

Garfinkel H (1967) *Studies in Ethnomethodology*, Prentice-Hall, Englewood Cliffs

Garfinkel H (1968) The origins of the term 'ethnomethodology', (excerpts) in *Ethnomethodology*, ed R Turner, Penguin, London, 15–18

General Medical Council (1993) *Professional Conduct and Discipline: Fitness to Practise*, GMC, London

Gervais KG (1986) *Redefining Death*, Yale University Press, New Haven

Giddens A (1976) *New Rules of Sociological Method*, Hutchinson and Co Ltd, London

Gillon R (1986) Conclusion: the Arthur case revisited. *British Medical Journal*, **292**, 543

Glasper A and Tucker A (eds) (1993) *Advances in Child Health Nursing*, Scutari Press, Harrow

Glover J (1970) *Responsibility*, Routledge and Kegan Paul, London

Goffman E (1967) *Interaction Ritual*, Penguin, Harmondsworth

Goldstone LA, Ball JA and Collier M (1983) *Monitor: an Index of the Quality of Nursing Care for Acute Medical and Surgical Wards*, Newcastle upon Tyne Polytechnic, Newcastle upon Tyne

Goodwin S, Dunford H and McNeill L (1991) One year on. *Community Outlook*, May, 17–18

Goulding J and Hunt J (1991) Accountability and legal issues in primary nursing, in *Primary Nursing in Perspective*, eds S Ersser and E Tutton, Scutari Press, London, 61–74

Green S (1992) Nurses cry freedom. *Health Service Journal*, 16 July, 21

Greenfield HI (1975) *Accountability in Health Facilities*, Praeger, New York

Grundstein-Amado R (1992) Differences in ethical decision-making processes among nurses and doctors. *Journal of Advanced Nursing*, **17**, 129–137

Grypdonk M (1987) *The Introduction of the Nursing Process in a Home Health Agency*. Paper presented at the International Nursing Research Congress, University of Edinburgh, July 29–30

Haldane E (1923) *The British Nurse in Peace and War*, Murray, London

Hall RH (1968) Professionalisation and bureaucratisation. *American Sociological Review*, **33**, 92–104

Hall RH (1969) *Occupations and the Social Structure*, Prentice Hall, New Jersey

Harré, R (1979) *Social Being*, Basil Blackwell, Oxford

Harré, R (1983) *Personal Being*, Basil Blackwell, Oxford

Harré, R and Gillett G (1994) *The Discursive Method*, Sage, London

Hartnett RT (1971) *Evaluation, Accountability and a Consideration of Some of the Problems of Assessing College Impact*, Educational Testing Service, Report No RM-71-1 Princeton University Press, Princeton, New Jersey

Harvey G (1991) An evaluation of approaches to assessing quality of nursing care using (predetermined) quality assurance tools. *Journal of Advanced Nursing*, **16**, 277–286

Healey P (1993) Arrangements for care. *Nursing Times*, **89**(3), 26–29

Hellema H (1992) Dutch issue guidelines on handicapped babies. *British Medical Journal*, **305**, 1312–1313

Helmstadter C (1993) Old nurses and new: nursing in the London teaching hospitals before and after the mid-nineteenth-century reforms. *Nursing History Review*, **1**, 43–70

Helson H (1964) *Adaptation Level Theory*, Harper and Row, London

Henderson V (1978) *The Nature of Nursing: a Definition and its Implications for Practice*, Macmillan, New York

Her Majesty's Government (1989) *The Children Act*, HMSO, London

Her Majesty's Government (1991) *Convention on the Rights of the Child Adopted by the General Assembly of the United Nations 20 November 1989*, HMSO, London

HMSO (1972) *Report of the Committee on Nursing* (The Briggs Report), HMSO, London

Hochschild AR (1983) *The Managed Heart: Commercialization of Human Feeling*, University of California Press, Berkeley

Hodgson J (1993) Employment law for nurses in *Central Health Studies series no. 6*, ed JH Tingle, Quay Press, Lancaster

Holden J, Sagovsky R and Cox JL (1989) Counselling in a general practice setting: controlled study of health visitor intervention in the treatment of postnatal depression. *British Medical Journal*, **298**, 223–226

House of Commons (1992) *Health Committee Second Report, Maternity Services*, HMSO, London

House of Lords (1993) *Airedale NHS Trust v Bland*, February 1993

Houston M and Weatherston L (1986) Creating change in midwifery: integrating theory and practice through practice-based research groups. *Midwifery*, **2**, 65–70

Hughes D (1980) *Lay Assessment of Clinical Seriousness*. PhD thesis, University of Swansea

Hughes D (1988) When nurse knows best: some aspects of nurse/doctor interaction in a casualty department. *Sociology of Health and Illness*, **10**, 1–22

Hugman J and McReady S (1993) Profiles make perfect practice. *Nursing Times*, **89**(27), 46–49

Humphries D (1978) *Jean's Way*, Quartet Books, London

Hunter D (1993) A sticking plaster job. *Health Service Journal*, 4 March, 28–29

Huntingdon J (1993) Nursing a buyer's instinct. *Health Services Journal*, 28 October, 19

Illich I (1977) *Limits to Medicine: Medical Nemesis. The Expropriation of Health*, Penguin, Harmondsworth

Institute of Medical Ethics Working Party (1990) Assisted death. *Lancet*, **336**, 610–613

Institute of Medical Ethics Working Party (1991) Withdrawal of life support from patients in a persistent vegetative state. *Lancet*, **337**, 96–98

International Council of Nurses (1965) *Code for Nurses*, ICN, Geneva

Isherwood K (1988) Friend or watchdog? *Nursing Times*, **84**(24), 65

Isherwood K (1989) Independent midwifery in the UK. *Midwife Health Visitor and Community Nurse*, **25**, 307–309

James A and Prout A (1990) *Constructing and Reconstructing Childhood: Contemporary Issues in the Sociological Study of Childhood*, Falmer Press, London

James JW (1979) Isabel Hampton and the professionalisation of nursing in the 1890s, in *The Therapeutic Revolution*, eds CE Rosenberg and MJ Vogel, University of Pennsylvania Press, Philadelphia, 201–244

Jennett B (1982) *High Technology Medicine: Benefits and Burdens*, Nuffield Provincial Hospital Trust, London

Johns C (1990) Autonomy of primary nurses: the need to both facilitate and limit autonomy in practice. *Journal of Advanced Nursing*, **15**, 886–894

Johns C (1991) Introducing and managing change – the move to primary nursing, in *Primary Nursing in Perspective*, eds S Ersser and E Tutton, Scutari Press, London, 31–48

Johns C (1993) Professional supervisor. *Journal of Nursing Management*, **1**, 9–18

Jones MA (1991) *Medical Negligence*, Sweet and Maxwell, London

Jones RM (ed) (1985) *Mental Health Act Manual*, Sweet and Maxwell, London

Kargar I (1992) Last chance for midwives. *Nursing Times*, **88**(24), 22

Kelleher A (1993) *Decisions, Decisions; A Talking Heads Booklet*, Broadcasting Support Services, London

Kitson A (1993) Quality and accountability (personal communication)

Kitzinger JV, Green JM and Coupland VA (1990) Labour relations: midwives and doctors on the labour ward, in *The Politics of Maternity Care: Services for Childbearing Women in the Twentieth Century*, eds J Garcia, R Kilpatrick and M Richards, Oxford University Press, Oxford, 149–162

Klein R and Redmayne S (1992) *Patterns of Priorities: a Study of the Purchasing and Rationing Policies of Health Authorities*. National Association of Health Authorities and Trusts (NAHAT) Research Paper No 7, NAHAT, Birmingham

Knowles D (1994) Accountability and commissioning. *KF News*, **17**(2), King's Fund, London, 1–2

Kramer M (1974) *Reality Shock: Why Nurses Leave Nursing*, Mosby, London

Kuhse H (1984) A modern myth. That letting die is not the intentional causation of death: some reflections on the trial and acquittal of Dr Leonard Arthur. *Journal of Applied Philosophy*, **1**, 21

Lamb D (1985) *Death, Brain Death and Ethics*, Croom Helm, London

Lanara V (1982) Responsibility in nursing. *International Nursing Review*, **29**, 7–10

Law Commission (1993) *Mentally Incapacitated Adults and Decision Making: Medical Treatment and Research.* Consultation paper No 129, HMSO, London

Leach MK (1993) Primary Nursing: autonomy or autocracy? *Journal of Advanced Nursing*, **18**, 394–400

Leadbetter S and Knight B (1993) Reporting deaths to coroners. *British Medical Journal*, **306**, 1018

Levine M (1990) Nursing ethics and the ethical nurse, in *Professional Ethics in Nursing*, eds L Thomson and H Thomson, Krieger, Malabar

Lewis FM and Batey MV (1982a) Clarifying autonomy and accountability in the nursing service, Part 1. *Journal of Nursing Administration*, **12**(9), 13–18

Lewis F. and Batey MV (1982b) Clarifying autonomy and accountability in nursing services, Part 2. *Journal of Nursing Administration*, **12**(10), 10–15

Lightfoot J, Baldwin S and Wright K (1992) *Nursing by Numbers?* Social Policy Research Unit and Centre for Health Economics, University of York

Linacre Centre Working Party (1982) *Euthanasia and Clinical Practice*, Linacre Centre, London

Lloyd GE (1969) *Aristotle: the Growth and Structure of His Thought*, Cambridge University Press, Cambridge

Loe R (1995) in *Nursing Law and Ethics*, eds JH Tingle and A Cribb, Blackwell Science, Oxford

Luckes EC (1914) *General Nursing*, Routledge and Kegan Paul, London

Lyman SM and Scott MB (1970) *A Sociology of the Absurd*, Appleton-Century-Crofts, New York

Macdonald AM (ed)(1981) *Chambers Twentieth Century Dictionary,* W and R Chambers, Edinburgh

MacIlwaine H (1980) *The Nursing of Female Neurotic Patients in Psychiatric Units of General Hospitals.* PhD thesis, University of Manchester

MacIlwaine H (1983) The communication patterns of female neurotic patients with nursing staff in psychiatric units of general hospitals, in *Nursing Research: Ten Studies of Patient Care*, ed J Wilson-Barnett, John Wiley and Sons, Chichester, 1–24

Mander R. (1986a) Refresher courses – unfulfilled potential? 1. *Midwives Chronicle and Nursing Notes*, **99**(1176), 4–5

Mander R (1986b) Refresher courses – unfulfilled potential? 2 *Midwives Chronicle and Nursing Notes*, **99**(1177), 39–41

Mander R (1992a) See how they learn: experience as the basis of practice. *Nurse Education Today*, **12**, 11–18

Mander R (1992b) Seeking approval for research access: the gatekeeper's role in facilitating a study of the care of the relinquishing mother. *Journal of Advanced Nursing*, **17**, 1460–1464

Mander R (1994) Autonomy, midwifery and maternity care. *Midwives Chronicle* (in press)

Manthey M (1980) *The Practice of Primary Nursing*, Blackwell, Boston

Manthey M (1991) Primary partners. *Nursing Times*, **87**(25), 27–28

Manthey M (1992) *The Practice of Primary Nursing*, (Revised edition), Kings Fund Centre, London

Marks IM, Hallam RS, Connoly J and Philpot R (1977) *Nursing in Behavioural Psychotherapy*, RCN, London

Marks P (1993) A community nursery nurse working with families with multiple births. *Health Visitor*, **66**(2), 56–58

Marr H and McCrae WA (1992) Multidisciplinary approach to standard setting (personal communication)

Mason JK and McCall-Smith RA (1994) *Law and Medical Ethics*, 4th edn, Butterworths, London

May D and Kelly MP (1982) Chancers, pests and poor wee souls: problems of legitimation in psychiatric nursing. *Sociology of Health and Illness*, **4**, 279–301

McClure ML (1984) Managing the professional nurse 2. Applying management theories to challenges. *Journal of Nursing Administration*, **14**, 11–17

McCormack B (1991) A case study identifying nursing staffs' perception of the delivery method of nursing care in practice on a particular ward. *Journal of Advanced Nursing*, **17**, 187–197

McGann S (1992) *The Battle of the Nurses*, Scutari Press, London

McHattie HE (1994) *Holding On?*, Books for Midwives Press, Cheshire

McHugh P (1968) *Defining the Situation*, Bobbs-Merrill, Indianapolis

McLymont M, Thomas S and Denham M (1986) *Health Visiting and the Elderly*, Churchill Livingstone, Edinburgh

McWhirter N (ed) *The Guinness Book of Records*, Bantam, New York

Mead D (1991) Defining primary nursing as a basis for comparison. *Nursing Times*, **87**(17), 71

MIDIRS (1992) Autonomy and accountability in midwifery. *MIDIRS Midwifery Database*, **12**

Miles K (1990) Health authority liable for negligent organisation of maternity services – Bull v. Devon Health Authority. Action for Victims of Medical Accidents. *Medical Legal Journal*, **11**, 11

Miles SH (1987) Futile feeding at the end of life: family virtues and treatment decisions. *Theoretical Medicine*, **8**, 293–302

Mollett Miss (1898) (Matron of the Royal South Hants Infirmary) The duty of the matron to her profession. *Nursing Record and Hospital World*, 25 June, 514

Morten H (1895) *How to Become a Nurse*, Scientific Press, London

Naughton B (1993) Funds of opportunity. *Nursing Times*, **89**(17), 62–64

Newdick C (1993) Rights to NHS resources after the 1990 Act. *Medical Law Review*, **1**, 53–82

Newson K (1986) Straight rules. *Nursing Times*, **82**(27), 19–20

NHS Management Executive Value for Money Unit (1993) *The Nursing Skill Mix in the District Nursing Service*, HMSO, London

Nursing Times (1921) 19 March, 313

Nuttall J (1993) *Punishment and Responsibility*, Polity Press, Cambridge

Old P (1993) HA law. *Health Service Journal*, 7 January, 21

Olsen DP (1992) Controversies in nursing ethics: a historical review. *Journal of Advanced Nursing*, **17**, 1020–1027

Orem DE (1991) *Nursing: Concepts of Practice*, Mosby, New York

Orr J (1993) Dangerous liaisons. *Health Visitor*, **66**, 27

Otter S (1990) *Learning Outcomes in Higher Education*, UDACE, London

Parker S and Wilson C (1992) *An Introduction to Medicolegal Aspects of Practice Nursing*, Medical Defence Union, London

Parsons T (1951) *The Social System*, Routledge and Kegan Paul, London

Passos J (1973) Accountability: myth or mandate? *Journal of Nursing Administration*, **3**, 17–22

Paterson J (1993) Leading role. *Nursing Times*, **89**(11), 59–60

Paton D and Brown R (1991) *Lifespan Health Psychology*, Harper Collins, London

Peachey M (1992) Practice makes perfect. *Nursing Times*, **88**(11), 59–60

Pearson A (1988) *Primary Nursing*, Croom Helm, London

Pearson A and Vaughan B (1986) *Nursing Models for Practice*, Heinemann Nursing, London

Pembrey S (1992) Understanding the relationship between the professional's autonomous role and their responsibility to the organisation, colleagues and patients. *Art and Science Seminar Series* (in press)

Peplau HE (1952) *Interpersonal Relations in Nursing*, GP Putnam, New York

Peplau HE (1971) Responsibility, authority, evaluation and accountability of nursing in patient care. *Michigan Nurse*, **44**, 20-23

Peplau H (1978) Psychiatric nursing: role of nurses and psychiatric nurses. *International Journal of Nursing Review*, **25**, 41–47

Percival RC (1970) Management of normal labour. *Practitioner*, **204**, 1221

Perry P (1990) Is there a need for a higher education inspectorate? in *Quality Assurance and Accountability in Higher Education*, ed C Loder, University of London Institute of Higher Education, London, 13–21

Phaneuf M (1976) *The Nursing Audit*, Appleton-Century-Crofts, New York

Pollock L (1989) *Community Psychiatric Nursing: Myth and Reality*, Scutari, Harrow

Potrykus C (1993) Public health role cut as GP contracts start to bite. *Health Visitor*, **66**, 188

Powell R (1991) *Measuring Performance in the Education of Adults: a Discussion Paper*, UDACE, London

Prentice S (1994) Accountability in the NHS. *KF News*, **17**(2), King's Fund, London, 2–3

Proud J (1988) Sound judgement. *Nursing Times*, **84**(29), 70–71

Pyne R (1992) *Understanding the Relationship Between the Professional's Autonomous Role and their Responsibility to Organisation, Colleagues and Patients*. Supervision of practice and research seminar, National Institute of Nursing, Oxford, 8 October

Queen Charlotte's College (1992) *Submission Document for the Validation of a Diploma/BSc (Hons) Higher Award*. (available from DMM)

Raffel S (1979) *Matters of Fact*, Routledge and Kegan Paul, London

Raman PG (1994) Let's return to learning. *The Independent*, 24 February

Re B. (1981) (A minor, wardship: medical treatment). *1 Weekly Law Report*, 1421

Re Claire C. Conroy (1985) 464 Atlantic 2nd 303 (New Jersey 1983) 486 Atlantic 2nd (New Jersey 1985)

Re J. (1990) (A minor, wardship: medical treatment). *3 All England Report 930* (1990) 2 Med Legal Report 67

Re J. (1992) Compelling a doctor to treat: Re J. a minor, medical treatment. *2 Family Law Reports*, 165

Re S. (1992) Adult: surgical treatment. *The Times Law Report*, 16 October

Regina v. Cambridge District Health Authority, *ex parte* B, (1995) *The Times Law Report*, 15 March

Reynolds W and Cormack D (1982) Clinical teaching: an evaluation of a problem oriented approach to psychiatric nurse education. *Journal of Advanced Nursing*, **7**, 231–237.

Reynolds W and Cormack D (1990) *Psychiatric and Mental Health Nursing: Theory and Practice*, Chapman & Hall, London

Riehl-Sisca JP (ed) (1989) *Conceptual Models for Nursing Practice*, Appleton and Lange, Norwalk CA

Ritter S (1989) *Bethlem and Maudsley Manual of Clinical Psychiatric Nursing Principles and Procedures*, Harper and Row, London

Ritter S (1992) Mental health legislation, in *A Textbook of Psychiatric and Mental Health Nursing*, eds JI Brooking, AH Ritter and BL Thomas, Churchill Livingstone, Edinburgh, 121–143

Robb IH (1909) An international education standard for nurses. *British Journal of Nursing*, 18 September, 233

Roberts L (1980) Primary nursing. *Canadian Nurse*, **76**(11), 20–23

Robinson DL (1971) Government contracting for academic research: accountability in the American experience, in *The Dilemma of Accountability in Modern Government*, eds BL Smith and DC Hague, Macmillan, New York, 103–117

Robinson S (1990) Maintaining the independence of the midwifery profession: a continuing struggle, in *The Politics of Maternity Care: Services for Childbearing Women in the Twentieth Century,* eds J Garcia, R Kilpatrick and M Richards, Oxford University Press, Oxford, 61–91

Robinson S, Golden J and Bradley S (1983) *A Study of the Role and Responsibilities of the Midwife.* Nursing Education Research Unit Report No 1; Kings College, University of London

Roch S (1988) Accountability in midwifery education. *Midwives Chronicle*, **101**(1205), 182–183

Roper N, Logan WW and Tierney AJ (1990) *The Elements of Nursing*, Churchill Livingstone, Edinburgh

Rowden R (1987) The UKCC code of conduct: accountability and implications. *Nursing*, **13**, 14

Roy C (1984) *Introduction to Nursing: an Adaptation Model*, Prentice Hall, London

Royal College of Nursing (1992) *Resuscitation: Right or Wrong? The Moral and Legal Issues Faced by Health Care Professionals*, RCN, London

Royal College of Nursing (1993a) *Dynamic Quality Improvement Programme – tutorial programme*, RCN, London

Royal College of Nursing (1993b) *Ethics Related to Research in Nursing*, Scutari Press, London

Royal College of Nursing Health Visitors' Advisory Group (1984) *Accountability in Health Visiting*, RCN, London

Royal College of Nursing Standards of Care Project (1990) *Quality Patient Care: the Dynamic Standard Setting System*, RCN, London

Rubington E and Weinberg MS (1987) *Deviance: the Interactionist Perspective*, 5th edn, Macmillan, New York

Russell B (1991) *The Problems of Philosophy*, Oxford University Press, Oxford

St John Smith P and Edwards LC (1992) Euthanasia. *British Medical Journal*, **305**, 1437

Salter B and Salter C (1993) Theatre of the absurd. *Health Service Journal*, 11 November, 30–31

Scheff T (1966) *Being Mentally Ill*, Aldine, Chicago

Schmitz P and O'Brien M (1986) Observations on nutrition and hydration in dying cancer patients, in *By No Extraordinary Means: the Choice to Forgo Life-Sustaining Food and Water*, ed J Lynn, Indiana University Press, Bloomington, 29–38

Schuetz A (1943) The problems of rationality in the social world. *Economica*, **10**, 130–179

Schuetz A (1943) The problem of responsibility in the social world. *Econometrica*, **10**, 130–149

Schutz A and Luckmann T (1974) *Structures of the Life World*, Heinemann, London

Seedhouse D (1986) *Health: the Foundations for Achievement*, Wiley, Chichester

Sewall MW (1905) How to lift your business into a profession (address to the Matrons' Council in London 1899: reprinted). *American Journal of Nursing*, **6**, 85–862

Shackleton J (1990) An achievement-led college, in *Assessment Debates*, ed T Horton, Hodder and Stoughton, London, 197–204

Shotter J (1984) *Social Accountability and Selfhood*, Basil Blackwell, Oxford

Shroeder PS and Maibusch RM (1984) *Nursing Quality Assurance. A Unit Based Approach*, Aspen, Rockville

Siler P (1986) Accountability on primary nursing emphasis. *Nursing*, **2**(1), 26–30

Smith DE (1978) 'K is mentally ill': the anatomy of a factual account. *Sociology*, **12**, 23–53

Smith G (1980) *Social Need*, Routledge and Kegan Paul, London

Smith JP (1981) Issues in nursing administration, in *Current Issues in Nursing*, ed L Hockley, Churchill Livingstone, Edinburgh, 64–78

Smith R (1991) Where is the wisdom...? the poverty of medical evidence. *British Medical Journal*, **303**, 798–799

Smith R (1992) Euthanasia: time for a Royal Commission. *British Medical Journal*, **305**, 728–729

Smith R (1993) The right to die. *EDIT: University of Edinburgh Magazine*, **3**, 8–10

SOHHD (1993) *Research and Development Strategy for the National Health Service in Scotland*, Chief Scientist Office, The Scottish Office Home and Health Department, Edinburgh

Stacey M (1976) The health service consumer: a sociological misconception. *Sociological Review*, **22**, 194–200

Steinbrook R and Lo B (1988) Artificial feeding – solid ground, not a slippery slope. *New England Journal of Medicine*, **318**, 286–290

Stevens B (1976) Accountability of the clinical specialist. *Journal of Nursing Administration*, **6**, 30–32

Stewart I (1895) A uniform curriculum of education for nurses. *Nursing Record and Hospital World*, 2 November, 311–313; 9 November, 330–332; 16 November, 349–351; and 23 November, 370–372

Stewart I (1898) The nursing conference, Miss Stewart's address. *Nursing Record and Hospital World*, 25 June, 512

Stewart I (1905) The twentieth century matron. *British Journal of Nursing*, 11 November, 392–396 and 18 November, 414–415

Stilwell R (1991) The rise of practice nursing. *Nursing Times*, **87**(24), 26–28

Stinson R and Stinson P (1983) *The Long Dying of Baby Andrew*, Little Brown and Company, New York

Styles M (1985) Accountable to whom? *International Nursing Review*, **32**, 73–75

Taylor M (1991) Unit power. *Health Visitor*, **64**, 238

Thompson IE, Melia KM, Boyd KM (1994) *Nursing Ethics*, 3rd edn, Churchill Livingstone, Edinburgh

Thompson JD (1967) *Organisations in Action*, McGraw Hill, New York

Tierney AJ and Taylor J (1991) Research in practice: an 'experiment' in researcher–practitioner collaboration. *Journal of Advanced Nursing*, **16**, 506–510

Tierney AJ, Taylor J, Closs SJ (1989) *A Study to Inform Nursing Support of Patients Coping With Chemotherapy for Breast Cancer*. Research Report, Nursing Research Unit, University of Edinburgh

Tierney AJ, Closs SJ, Hunter HC and Macmillan MS (1993) Experiences of elderly patients concerning discharge from hospital. *Journal of Clinical Nursing*, **2**, 179–185

Tilley S (1995) *Negotiating Realities*, Avebury Press, Aldershot

Tilley S (in press) Notes on narrative knowledge in psychiatric nursing. *Journal of Psychiatric and Mental Health Nursing*

Tingle JH (1990a) A duty of care. *Nursing Times*, **86**(30), 60–61

Tingle JH (1990b) Ethics in practice. *Nursing Times*, **86**(48), 54–55

Tingle JH (1990c) Accountability and the law: how it affects the nurse. *Senior Nurse*, **10**(2), 8–9

Tingle JH (1991) Negligence: the new accountability. *Nursing Standard*, **5**(29), 18–19

Tingle JH (1992a) Some legal issues in wound management. *Nursing Standard*, **6**(34), 4–6

Tingle JH (1992b) Court in the slips. *Health Service Journal*, 20–22

Tingle JH (1992c) Primary nursing and the law. *British Journal of Nursing*, **1**, 248–251

Tingle JH (1993a) The extended role of the nurse: legal implications. *Care of the Critically Ill*, **9**, 30–34

Tingle JH (1993c) Legal and professional implications of the named nurse concept. *British Journal of Nursing*, **2**, 480–482

Tingle JH and Cribb A (eds) (1995) *Nursing Law and Ethics*, Blackwell Science, Oxford

Towell D (1975) *Understanding Psychiatric Nursing*, Royal College of Nursing, London

Tschudin V (1989) *Ethics in Nursing: the Caring Relationship*, Heinemann Nursing, Oxford

Tschudin V (1992) *Ethics in Nursing*, 2nd edn, Butterworth Heinemann, Oxford

Turner BS (1987) *Medical Power and Social Knowledge,* Sage, London

Twinn S (1991) Conflicting paradigms of health visiting practice: a continuing debate for professional practice. *Journal of Advanced Nursing*, **16**, 966–973

Twinn S, Dauncey J and Carnell J (1990) *The Process of Health Profiling*, Health Visitors' Association, London

Uden G, Norberg A, Lindseth A and Marhaug V (1992) Ethical reasoning in nurses' and physicians' stories about care episodes. *Journal of Advanced Nursing*, **127**, 1028–1034

UKCC (1989) *Exercising Accountability*, United Kingdom Central Council for Nursing, Midwifery and Health Visiting, London

UKCC (1992a) *Code of Professional Conduct*, 3rd edn, United Kingdom Central Council for Nursing, Midwifery and Health Visiting, London

UKCC (1992b) *The Scope of Professional Practice*, United Kingdom Central Council for Nursing, Midwifery and Health Visiting, London

UKCC (1993) *Standards for Records and Record Keeping*, United Kingdom Central Council for Nursing, Midwifery and Health Visiting, London

Unsworth C (1987) *The Politics of Mental Health Legislation*, Clarendon Press, Oxford

Utley A (1992) Good intentions, fatal outcomes. *Times Higher Education Supplement*, 2 October, 44

Vaughan B (1989) Autonomy and accountability. *Nursing Times*, **85**(3), 54–55

Vincent JL (1990) European attitudes towards ethical problems in intensive care medicine: results of an ethical questionnaire. *Intensive Care Medicine*, **16**, 256–264

Wade B (1993) The job satisfaction of health visitors, district nurses and practice nurses working in areas served by four trusts: year 1. *Journal of Advanced Nursing*, **18**, 992–1004

Walker J (1976) Midwife or obstetric nurse? Some perceptions of midwives and obstetricians of the role of the midwife. *Journal of Advanced Nursing*, **1**, 129–138

Walker J (1972) The changing role of the midwife. *International Journal of Nursing Studies*, **9**, 85–94

Wandelt M and Ager J (1974) *Quality Patient Care Scale*, Appleton-Century-Crofts, New York

Watson R (1992) Justifying your practice. *Nursing*, **5**(3), 11–13

Watson R (1994) Practical ethical aspects of the care of patients with dementia. *Nursing Ethics*, **1**(3), 181–192

While A and Rees K (1993) The knowledge base of health visitors and district nurses regarding products in the proposed formulary for nurse prescription. *Journal of Advanced Nursing*, **18**, 1573–1577

White R (1977) Accountability – a necessity for survival? *Nursing Mirror*, 17 November, 25

Williams G and Loder C (1990) The importance of quality and quality assurance, in *Quality Assurance and Accountability in Higher Education*, ed C Loder, University of London Institute of Higher Education, London, 1–12

Williams S, Calnan M, Cants S and Coyle J (1993) All change in the NHS? Implications of the NHS reforms for primary care prevention. *Sociology of Health and Illness*, **15**, 43–67

Wilson-Barnett J and Fordham M (1982) *Recovery from Illness*, John Wiley, London

Wood C (1901) A retrospect and a forecast. Transactions of the Third International Congress of Nurses Pan-American Exposition, Buffalo, 18–21 September, 374

Wooff K and Goldberg D (1988) Further observations on the practice of community care in Salford: differences between community psychiatric nurses and mental health social workers. *British Journal of Psychiatry*, **153**, 30–37

World Health Organization (1978) *Alma Ata Declaration*, WHO, Copenhagen

World Health Organization (1986) *Charter for Health Promotion*, WHO/Canadian Public Health Alliance, Ottowa

Wright SG (1991) Of primary importance. *Nursing Times*, **87**(10), 38–41

Zander K (1988) Nursing care management; strategic management of cost and quality outcomes. *Journal of Nursing Administration*, **18**, 23–30

Index

Ability
  necessary for accountability 70,
    149–50
  of primary nurses 75
  see also Knowledge
Accountability
  definitions 2, 33, 49, 84, 96, 97, 124,
    167–8, 212
  factors in achieving 60, 70
Accountability in Health Visiting (RCN
    document) 139
Accounting (making statements of
    behaviour), in psychiatric nursing
  vs accounts 119
  formal and informal 119–20
  a form of labour 119
  a system of discipline 120
  systems of power 120–2
  templates for 123–4
Accounts (statements of behaviour), in
    psychiatric nursing
  vs accounting 119
  classification of 114–16
  and competence 111–13
  a form of social practice 109
  in the form of stories 113
  making actions observable 109–10
  neglect of common sense 111
  not a theoretical framework 111
  patients' 114–16
  perspectives of 109–10
  and professional judgement 113–14,
    116
  template accounts 117–19
  and working ideologies 116–17
Action for Sick Children (ASC) 154–5
Activities of living model of nursing

  (Roper, Logan and Tierney) 41–2
Adaptation model of nursing (Roy's)
    39–40
Administrative authority 53
Advisory Group on Nurse Prescribing 140
Advocacy 170–1
Aristotle 149–50, 154
ASC (Action for Sick Children) 154–5
Assessment, in the nursing process 41–2
Assisted death
  arguments against 192–4
  arguments for 190–2
  case of Dr Nigel Cox 183–4
  ethical considerations 182–5, 203–5
  and the law 186–7
  in neonatal care 201–2
  nurses' attitudes to 181–2
  and patient autonomy 182–3
  see also Death; Euthanasia; Feeding;
    Resuscitation; Treatment
Associate nurses, role in primary nursing
    88
Audit
  audit committee 60
  authority for nurses to carry out 60
  clinical 60–1
  of community nursing records 142
  definition 60, 142
  see also Quality assurance; Standards;
    Standard setting
Authority
  administrative 53
  and autonomy 53–4
  definition 54
  of expert knowledge 52–3
  freedoms needed for 148
  in paediatric nursing 153–5

Authority *contd*
positional 53
prerequisite for accountability 70
in primary nursing 75, 80–1
situational 53
sources of 52–3
in traditional nursing 84–5
Autonomy
accountability as consequence of 54
attitudinal 53, 102
and authority 53–4
of children 152–3
definitions 53, 54, 101
and midwifery 101–4
nurses vs other health-care
professionals 84
patient autonomy 83, 195
personal 102
in primary nursing 75, 83–4
of research participants 219
and standard setting 62, 63
structural 53, 102
work-related 53

Babies, handicapped, *see* Neonatal care
Beneficence 178, 179
Biculturalism, in education 238
alternatives to 238
Bland, Tony 184–5
BNA, *see* British Nurses' Association
BPA (British Paediatricians
Association) 155
BRCS (British Red Cross Society) 26
Briggs Committee 210
British Journal of Nursing 23
British Nurses' Association (BNA)
campaign for nurse registration 20–1
and educational needs 20–1
founding of 18, 19
see also Royal British Nurses'
Association
British Paediatricians Association (BPA)
155
British Red Cross Society (BRCS) 26
Budgets, accountability for 3–4
Bull vs Devon Area Health Authority
172–3
Bureaucracy, and primary nursing 71, 78–9

Care
accountability becoming remote from
delivery 35
continuity of, in primary nursing 74–6
holistic, in primary nursing 81–3
legal duty of 164, 171
patient-centred, in primary nursing
75–6
see also Negligence; Nursing
Care plans, in primary nursing 74
Caring, commitment to 193, 204
Case discussions, in community care 144
Case managers 91
Case meetings, in primary nursing 86
Case method, *see* Patient allocation
Central Committee for the State
Registration of Nurses 25, 27
Change
accountability as vehicle for 47
managers' recommendations for 48
Charge nurses, role in primary nursing
77–9, 85, 88
Children
autonomy of 152–3
knowledge of impending death 152–3
loss of innocence 159
responsibility for treatment of 156
responsibility of 158–60
self-medication 152
shared accountability 149
as small adults 148–9
see also Paediatric nursing; Parents
Clinical audit 60–1
Code of Professional Conduct (UKCC)
aims of 212
collaboration with other health-care
professionals 225
and commercial considerations 215–16
confidentiality 220
as guide to practice 180
inappropriate delegation 145
major accountability to patients 51
and nurse researchers 212
nurses' knowledge of 188
patients' condition and safety 188,
218–19
patients' interests and wellbeing 188,
218

privileged position and relationship 219
provision of patient care 170
requirement to practise according to 33
and standards of practice 188
Colleagues, accountability to 169
College of Health 67
College of Nursing 27
Community concept of 131
Community Health Councils 67
Community nurses
  'advanced practitioner' proposals 140–1
  cooperation with other workers 131
  delegation of authority 135
  growing amount of administration 134
  health profiling 136–7
  NHS reforms 132–3
  as providers 132
  record keeping 141–2
  responsibility to community 131
  see also Community nursing; District nurses; Health visitors; Practice nurses
Community nursing
  case study 143–5
  legal and professional issues in 138
  NHS and Community Care Act (1990) 137, 138
  overview 11
  patient participation in care 143
  prerequisites for practice 139
  and Project 2000 135–6
  resource allocation 134
  responsibility and accountability 138
  skill mix 134
  team work 139
  see also Community nurses
Compensation, role of the law 164, 165
Complaints system, in midwifery 106
Confidentiality, in research projects 220–1, 224
Conscientious objection 196
Consent
  for research 217–18
  of research participants 219
Consultants, relationships with junior doctors 55

Continuity of care, in primary nursing 74–6
Court cases
  Bull vs Devon Area Health Authority 172–3
  Knight and Others vs Home Office and Another 173–4
  obligation to treat 174–5
  and resource allocation 172–6
Cox, Dr Nigel 183–4

Death
  need to rethink attitudes to 204
  nurses' attitude to 181–2
  survival greater disaster than 204
  see also Assisted death; Dying; Life and death decisions
Decision making
  decentralization in primary nursing 80–1
  see also Life and death decisions
Delegation of responsibilities
  in community nursing 135, 145
  in primary nursing 75
Deterrence, as function of law 165
Diagnosis, mistaken 193–4
Disciplinary power 127
Disclosure
  and accountability 96
  in clinical audit 61
  definition 50
  in external regulation 54
  formal 54
  guidelines for 54
  in internal regulation 55
  to patients 67
  vs recounting 49
  referent others 50–1, 55
  responsibility for initiation 50
Disputes, role of the law in resolution 164–5
Distributive justice 191–2, 196
District nurses
  assessment by 135
  and nurse prescribing 140
  time spent on administration 134
District nursing, NHS Management Executive review of skill mix 134

Dock, Lavinia 22
Doctors, junior, relationships with
    consultants 55
Documentation
    in communicating decisions 40–1
    in nursing evaluation 46
    see also Records
Drugs, intravenous, authority to administer
    52
Dutch Society of Paediatrics 201–2
Dying
    prisoners of technology 190–1
    see also Assisted death; Death
Dynamic standard-setting system 57, 58,
    62, 64

Economic and Social Research Council
    (ESRC) 215
Education and training
    19th century need for standardization
      20
    accountability in 232–4
    achievement-led outcome-based
      learning 235–6
    apprenticeship training system 29
    biculturalism in 238
    course planning and delivery 234–5
    demonstration of accountability 234
    differing methods of 36
    English National Board (ENB) 36
    as function of law 166
    higher education 233, 235–6
    nurses' role in 44
    outcomes 235–6
    overview 16–17
    for primary nursing 76–7
    purchaser–provider split 233–4
    reflective activities 239
    refresher courses for midwives 104
    responsibilities of nurse educationalists
      150
    role modelling 239
    standard setting 237
    teaching and learning accountability
      239
    theoretical and clinical base 237
    validation, monitoring and review
      236–7

    see also Health education; Project 2000
Employee accountability 168
English National Board (ENB) 36
Errors, see Mistakes
Ethical Guidelines for Nursing Research
    (RCN document) 220, 224–5, 229
Ethics 177–80
    and assisted death 182–5, 203–5
    morality vs legality 186
    and nursing research 216–18
    overview 13
    principles of 216–17
    see also Code of Professional Conduct
Eugenics 191
Euthanasia 182, 186
    active vs passive 191
    in the Netherlands 182
    see also Assisted death
Evaluation
    accountability as form of 66
    formative 45
    in the nursing process 45–6
    summative 46
Exercising Accountability (UKCC
    guidelines) 108
Expert Maternity Group 141–2

Family 4, 169
    see also Parents
Feeding
    artificial, constitutes treatment 198
    case of Tony Bland 184–5
    case study 197–200
    differing perceptions of 199
    withdrawal of 199
Fenwick, Mrs Bedford
    and College of Nursing 27
    expulsion from RBNA 22
    founder member of BNA 20
    founder of Matrons' Council 22
    and Select Committee 24
Fiduciary responsibility 179
Free will 154
Fundholding practices, scope for primary
    health care 133
Funding, of research, see Sponsors

'Gatekeepers' in research, see Research
    'gatekeepers'

General Nursing Council (GNC) 20, 24, 25, 28
General practitioners (GPs), new NHS contracts 132
GNC (General Nursing Council) 20, 24, 25, 28
Goal setting, in the nursing process 42–3
GPs, *see* General practitioners
Grants for research, *see* Sponsors
Great War (World War I) 26–7

HA (Hospitals Association) 19
Harm, duty to avoid 195–6
Health-care assistants (HCAs) 81–2
Health education 44
Health profiling 136–7
Health visitors
    advocacy role 143
    assessment by 135
    lack of recognition 135
    NHS reforms and 133
    and nurse prescribing 140
    time spent on administration 134
    uncovering health needs 137
Heathrow Debate 2
Hierarchies
    diminishing midwives' accountability 99
    hierarchical accountability 54, 55–6
    midwives' 101
    of responsibility 71
    and standard setting 63
Hippocratic Oath 187
Hospitals
    changing 19th century perceptions of 19
    dependent on nurse training schools 29
Hospitals Association (HA) 19

ICN (International Council of Nurses) 23
Incompetent patient, case study 200–2
Institutional accountability
    of midwives 98–9
    in psychiatric nursing 107–8
Interactionist model of nursing (Riehl's) 42, 43–4
International Congress of Women (1899) 22–3

International Council of Nurses (ICN) 23
Intervention, central part of nursing process 43–5
Intravenous drugs, authority to administer 52

Judgement, of patient, impaired 194
Justice, *see* Distributive justice

Key workers 91
Knight and Others vs Home Office and Another 173–4
Knowledge
    authority of 52–3
    as base for accountability 35–6
    basis for decision making 44
    dangers of underestimation of 43
    in specialty areas 36
    see also Ability; Nursing research

Law
    affects all aspects of nursing 166–7
    and assisted death 186–7
    and compensation 164, 165
    conflicts of interest 164
    criminal 165
    deterrent function 165
    education function 166
    establishing negligence 164–5
    ignorance of is no excuse 163
    legality vs morality 186
    personal injury actions 165
    regulation function 165–6
    resolution of disputes 164–5
    respect for medical judgement 175
    role of 164
    vicarious liability 165
    see also Court cases; Legal accountability
League of St Bartholomew's Nurses 23
Legal (legislative) accountability 169, 171
    employees could be directly liable 171
    of midwives 100–1
    overview 12–13
    vs professional accountability 18
    of psychiatric nurses 125
    see also Court cases; Law
Legal issues, in community nursing 138

Liability
  responsibility as form of 157
  see also Vicarious liability
Life
  sanctity of 186, 192–3
  see also Neonatal care; Quality of life
Life and death decisions
  in neonatal care 201–2
  overview 13–15
  see also Assisted death; Euthanasia
Literature, legal aspects of failing to read
      166
Luckes, Eva 21, 24, 28

Managers
  accountability to patients 71
  perception of accountability 47, 142
  in primary nursing 88–9
  ratification and support from 47, 63
Maternity care 142
  negligence in, court case 172–3
Matrons' Council of Great Britain and
      Ireland 22–3
Maturity, *see* Professional maturity
Medical press, legal aspects of failing to
      read 166
Medical Research Council (MRC) 215
Medical staff
  relationships in primary nursing 79–80
  see also Consultants; Doctors
Mental Health Act (1983) 125
Midwifery
  autonomy in 101–4
  close association with nursing 105
  medical practitioners in 105
  non-implementation of research-based
      knowledge 104–5
  overview 9–10
  team midwifery 105
  vicarious liability in 106
Midwives
  accountability to the mother 99
  compared with obstetricians 102–3
  and complaints system 106
  hierarchy of accountability 101
  implications of accountability 106
  institutional accountability 98–9
  legislative accountability 100–1

'obstetric nurses' 98
personal accountability 99–100
prerequisites for accountabiiity 104–5
tasks appropriate to 103
Midwives Act (1902) 24, 100
Midwives' Rules 100
Mistakes
  dealing with, in primary nursing 86–7
  impaired judgement 194
  mistaken diagnosis 193–4
  primary vs traditional nursing 87
Models of nursing
  and accountability 39
  focus on knowledge base 34
  Orem's self-care model 38, 44, 45–6
  overview 6
  Peplau's model 34, 42
  perceptions of 38
  Riehl's interactionist model 42, 43–4
  Roper, Logan and Tierney activities of
      living model 41–2
  Roy's adaptation model 39–40
  see also Nursing process
Monitor (QA tool) 58
Moral accountability 217–18
Morality
  individual vs professional 180
  vs legality 186
Multiple accountability 4–5

Named nurses 73, 89, 91
National Association for the Welfare of
      Children in Hospital (NAWCH)
      154–5
National Council of Nurses 23
National Council of Trained Nurses 26
National Health Service (NHS)
  extending primary care role 132
  reforms 132
  as source of research funding 215
  see also entries beginning with NHS
National Health Service Training
      Department (NHSTD) 236
NAWCH (National Association for the
      Welfare of Children in Hospital)
      154–5
Negligence
  court cases 172–4

establishing 164–5
and reading of journal articles 166
Neonatal care, life and death decisions
    201–2
NHS, *see* National Health Service
NHS and Community Care Act (1990),
    and community nursing 137, 138
NHS Management Executive (NHSME),
    review on skill mix in district
    nursing 134
NHS Trusts, attitudes to research 223
Nightingale, Florence 21, 28
Nurse–patient relationship, in psychiatric
    nursing 108
Nurse prescribing 105, 140
Nurse researchers
    accountability to
        co-researchers 225–6
        'gatekeepers' 221–2, 224–5
        participants 218–21
        research ethics committees 216–18
        sponsors 214–16
        the public 227–8
    autonomy of 213, 214
    and commercial considerations 215–16
    dual role of 211–12, 228–30
    moral accountability 217–18
    professional accountability 226–7
    tensions of multiple accountability
        228–30
    and the UKCC Code of Professional
        Conduct 212
    to whom accountable 214
    see also Nursing research
Nurses
    conflict of accountability 170–1
    early apathy towards registration 25
    educative role 44
    formal vs informal accountability
        124–5
    lack of homogeneity 105
    limitation of accountability 127–8
    management of accountability 126–7
    mobilization in World War I 26
    prescribing 105, 140
        primary accountability to patients 51
        role in resource allocation 170–1
        suspicion of accountability 37

to whom accountable 3–4, 168–9
see also Charge nurses; Community
    nurses; District nurses; Health
    visitors; Midwives; Named nurses;
    Nurse researchers; Nursing;
    Practice nurses; Psychiatric nurses;
    Registration
Nurses Registration Act (1919) 27–8
Nursing
    all aspects affected by the law 166–7
    ambiguity about future 34–5
    complicated nature of accountability in
        4
    historical overview 5–6
    history 18–19
    line management culture 177–8
    organization of 177–8
    professional features of 3
    replacement of doer by supervisor 35
    traditional structure 77, 84
    see also Care; Community nursing;
        Nurses; Paediatric nursing; Patient
        allocation; Primary nursing;
        Professionalism; Psychiatric
        nursing; Task allocation; Team
        nursing
Nursing assistants 81–2
Nursing models, *see* Models of nursing
Nursing process
    able to be justified 41
    assessment 41–2
    circular or spiralling process 40
    evaluation 45–6
    intervention 43–5
    overview 6–7
    planning and goal setting 42–3
    a problem-solving approach 34, 40
    stages in 40
    see also Models of nursing
Nursing research
    accountability in 211–14
    in an accountable profession 209–11
    confidentiality in 220–1, 224
    consent for 217–18
    consent of participants 219
    definition 210–11
    DoH strategies 210, 211, 227
    ethical 216–17

gap between research and practice
226–7
growth of 210
increasing scrutiny and regulation
213–14
multidisciplinary research 225–6
need in midwifery 104–5
and nurses' accounting 122–3
nurses as researchers 211–12
overview 15–16
RCN ethical guidelines 220, 224–5,
229
scope for, in primary nursing 73–4
see also Knowledge; Nurse
researchers; Sponsors

Obligations *see* Responsibility
Obstetricians
compared with midwives 102–3
increase in numbers and power of 98
Orem's self-care model 38, 44, 45–6

Paediatric nursing
authority in 153–5
definition 148
involving parents 150–2
overview 12
political activism 150, 154–5
Project 2000 nurses 148
responsibility in 155–60
shared accountability 149
see also Children; Parents
Paediatrics, Dutch Society of Paediatrics
201–2
PAP (principle of alternative possibilities)
156
Parents
accountability for children's welfare
151–2
involvement in paediatric nursing
150–2
responsibility for children's treatment
156
responsibility of 158–60
shared accountability 149
see also Children; Family; Paediatric
nursing

Participants in research, *see* Research
participants
Partnerships
in community nursing 144–5
in primary nursing 81–2
Pastoral power 127
Patient advocacy 170–1
Patient allocation 75, 77
Patient autonomy
and continuation of treatment 195
in primary nursing 83
Patients
accountability to 51, 168
autonomy of, in primary nursing 83–4
major line of nurses' accountability 51
nurses' accountability to or for 4
participation in community care 143
role in standard setting and quality
assurance 65–6, 67
self-interpretation 127
see also Nurse–patient relationship
Patients' Association 67
Peer review 60
Peer support, in primary nursing 79
Peplau's model of nursing 34, 42
Personal accountability, of midwives
99–100
Phaneuf Nursing Audit 58
Planning of care, in the nursing process
42–3
Pluralistic accountability, in primary
nursing 84
Political activism, in paediatric nursing
150, 154–5
Positional authority 53
Post-registration education and practice
(PREP) 140
Power
disciplinary 127
pastoral 127
and political action 154–5
from standard setting 59–60
Practice nurses
growth in numbers 139
health profiling 136–7
lack of appropriate training 140
PREP (post-registration education and
practice) 140

Prescribing, by nurses 105, 140
Primary nurses
    abilities of 75
    authority of 80–1
    partnership with health-care and
        nursing assistants 81–2
    see also Primary nursing
Primary nursing
    accountability, levels of 88
    accountability in 71, 75, 84–9, 89–91
    associate nurse role 88
    authority in 75
    autonomy in 75, 83–4
    benefits of 91
    and bureaucracy 71, 78–9
    case meetings 86
    charge nurse role 77–9, 85, 88
    collegial system 81
    continuity of care 74–6
    dealing with mistakes 86–7
    decision making decentralization 80–1
    definition 74
    education and preparation 76–7
    features of 71–2, 74
    health-care assistant role 81, 81–2
    holistic care 81–3
    inter-team conflict 79–80
    key elements in 74, 75
    legal dangers in 24-hour accountability
        90
    management role 88–9
    overview 8–9
    patient autonomy in 83
    peer support 79
    pluralistic accountability 84
    referent others in 55
    relations with medical staff 79
    responsibility in 75, 76, 87–8
    rising popularity of 72–4
    roles in 55
    scope for research in 73–4
    structure of 77
    team meetings 86
    see also Primary nurses
Principle of alternative possibilities (PAP)
    156
Professional accountability 169
    vs legal accountability 18

in life and death decisions 187–90
    in research 226–7
Professionalism
    and accountability 2–3, 4–5, 18
    through accountability 33, 34, 36
    emergence of 18–19
    progress before World War I 23–4
    see also Professional accountability;
        Professional maturity; Registration
        of nurses
Professional maturity
    and accountability 37
    definition 35
    involvement of others 37
    knowledge and 35–6
    teamwork 36–7
Professional responsibility, see
    Responsibility
Professionals, perception of accountability
    142
Project 2000 34–5
    community nurses 135–6
    paediatric nurses 148
    student training in the community
        135–6
Psychiatric nurses
    and accountability 107–9
    accountable to researchers and
        professionalizers 108
    formal and informal authority 124–5
    inability to account for practice 108–9
    institutional accountability 107–8
    legal accountability 125
    see also Psychiatric nursing
Psychiatric nursing
    management of accountability 126–7
    models of 128–9
    nurse–patient relationship 108
    overview 10
    see also Accounting; Accounts;
        Psychiatric nurses
Public, accountability of researchers to
    227–8

Quality assurance (QA)
    employee involvement 58
    to identify opportunities for
        improvement 58, 66

method of achieving accountability 65–8
outcomes 61–2, 65
patients' role in 67
practitioner-based 63, 66
recounting in 58
to remove poor performers 57–8, 66–7
tools 58
varied experiences of 58
see also Audit; Standards; Standard setting
Quality of life 196–7
in treating neonates 201
Qualpacs 58
Queen Alexandra's Imperial Military Nursing Service 26

RBNA, see Royal British Nurses' Association
Records
aids to evaluation and research 179
in community nursing 141–2
confidentiality of 220
in nursing evaluation 46
see also Documentation
Recounting
definition 50
vs disclosure 49
in quality assurance 58
Referent others (in disclosure) 50–1
in primary nursing 55
Reflection, as accountability learning tool 239
Registration, of nurses
abroad 24
BNA campaign 20–1
early apathy of nurses 25
early parliamentary bills 24–5
impact of World War I 26–7
international aspects 23–4
Nurses Registration Act (1919) 27–8
political considerations 28
RBNA charter setback 21
supplementary registers 28
Regulation
external 54, 55–6, 68
as function of law 165–6
internal 55, 68

internalization of accountability 68
move towards internal mechanisms 56–7
Relatives 4, 169
see also Parents
Research, see Nursing research
Research and Development Strategy 211
Researchers, see Nurse researchers
Research ethics committees 216–18
Research 'gatekeepers'
accountability of researchers to 221–2, 224–5
changing relationships with researchers 223–4
procedures 222–3
reports for 224
Research participants
accountability of researchers to 218–21
dependence of 218
respecting autonomy 219
respecting confidentiality 220–1, 224
Resource allocation
in community nursing 134
and continuation of treatment 196
court cases 172–6
distributive justice 191–2
nurses' role in 170–1
Respect for persons 178–9
Responsibility
avoidance of 157
in community nursing 138
consequences of 157–8
definition 51, 155
fiduciary 179
a form of liability 157
levels of 179–80
of nurse educationalists 150
in paediatric nursing 155–60
of parents and children 158–60
personal 179
prerequisite for accountability 70
in primary nursing 75, 76, 87–8
principle of alternative possibilities (PAP) 156
for professional practice 179–80
realms of 179–80
to society 180
for treatment of children 156

see also Delegation
Responsibility barter game 157, 158, 159
Resuscitation
case study 194–7
position documents 188
Riehl's interactionist model of nursing 42, 43–4
Rights, considerations in life and death decisions 190
Robb, Isabel Hampton 22
Role modelling 239
Roper, Logan and Tierney activities of living model of nursing 41–2
Royal British Nurses' Association (RBNA)
control gained by opponents of registration 21
and register of nurses 21
see also British Nurses' Association
Royal College of Nursing (RCN)
Accountability in Health Visiting 139
dynamic standard-setting system 57, 58, 62, 64
Ethical Guidelines for Nursing Research 220, 224–5, 229
Paediatric Society 155
Research Committee 227
Roy's adaptation model of nursing 39–40

Sanctions, for professional transgression 169
Scope of Professional Practice 52, 135, 140
Self-accountability 169
Self-care model of nursing (Orem's) 38, 44, 45–6
Self-concept, in Roy's adaptation model of nursing 40
Self-determination, *see* Autonomy
Sewall, May Wright 22, 23
Situational authority 53
Skill mix, in community nursing 134
Slippery slope 193
Society accountability 169
Society for the State Registration of Nurses 24
Sponsors, of research
accountability of researchers to 214, 215–16

commercial organizations 215–16
contracts with 215, 216
reports for 215
sources of sponsorship 214–15
Standards
definition 57
formulation of 57–8
overview 7–8
practitioner–based 64
ratification of nurses' 63
triple function in patient care 64
see also Audit; Quality assurance; Standard setting
Standard setting
and autonomy 62, 63
dynamic standard-setting system 57, 58, 62, 64
in education 237
educational function 64
involvement of patients 67–8
literature search in 65
patients' role in 65–6
power in 59–60
practitioner-based approach 59
responsibility for 59
unit-based approach 58
see also Audit; Quality assurance; Standards
Stewart, Isla 20, 22, 24
Strategy for Research in Nursing, Midwifery and Health Visiting 210, 227
Suicide 186
Supervision 55
Supervisor of Midwives 100–1
Support
environment of 47
from peers, in primary nursing 79

Task allocation 72, 75
Team meetings, in primary nursing 86
Team midwifery 105
Team nursing 64, 72–3, 75
Teamwork 36
collaboration in 36–7, 196
in community nursing 139
in research 225–6
Technology, extending life 190–1

Training, *see* Education and training
Treatment
  consideration of alternatives 196
  constraints on 195–6
  determining advisability of 197
  obligation to treat, legal aspects 174–5
  refusal of 186–7
  withholding 186–7, 202–3

United Kingdom Central Council for
    Nursing, Midwifery and Health
    Visiting (UKCC)
  accountability to 168
  Exercising Accountability (guidelines)
    108
  post-registration education and practice
    (PREP) 140
  and professional regulation 51
  Scope of Professional Practice 52, 135,
    140

see also Code of Professional Conduct
Utilitarianism 180

VADs (BRCS Voluntary Aid Detachment
    members) 26
Vegetative states
  case of Tony Bland 184–5
  case study 197–200
Vicarious liability 165
  in midwifery 106
Volunteer untrained nurses in World War I
    26

War (World War I) 26–7
WHO (World Health Organization), health
    targets 132, 133
Wood, Catherine 22
World Health Organization (WHO), health
    targets 132, 133
World War I 26–7